Feed Your Health 2

Over 100 delicious,
healthy recipes

Alli Godbold

Published by New Generation Publishing in 2019

Copyright © Alli Godbold 2019

First Edition

The author asserts the moral right under the Copyright, Designs and Patents Act 1988 to be identified as the author of this work.

All Rights reserved. No part of this publication may be reproduced, stored in a retrieval system or transmitted, in any form or by any means without the prior consent of the author, nor be otherwise circulated in any form of binding or cover other than that which it is published and without a similar condition being imposed on the subsequent purchaser.

ISBN: 978-1-78955-701-5

www.newgeneration-publishing.com

New Generation Publishing

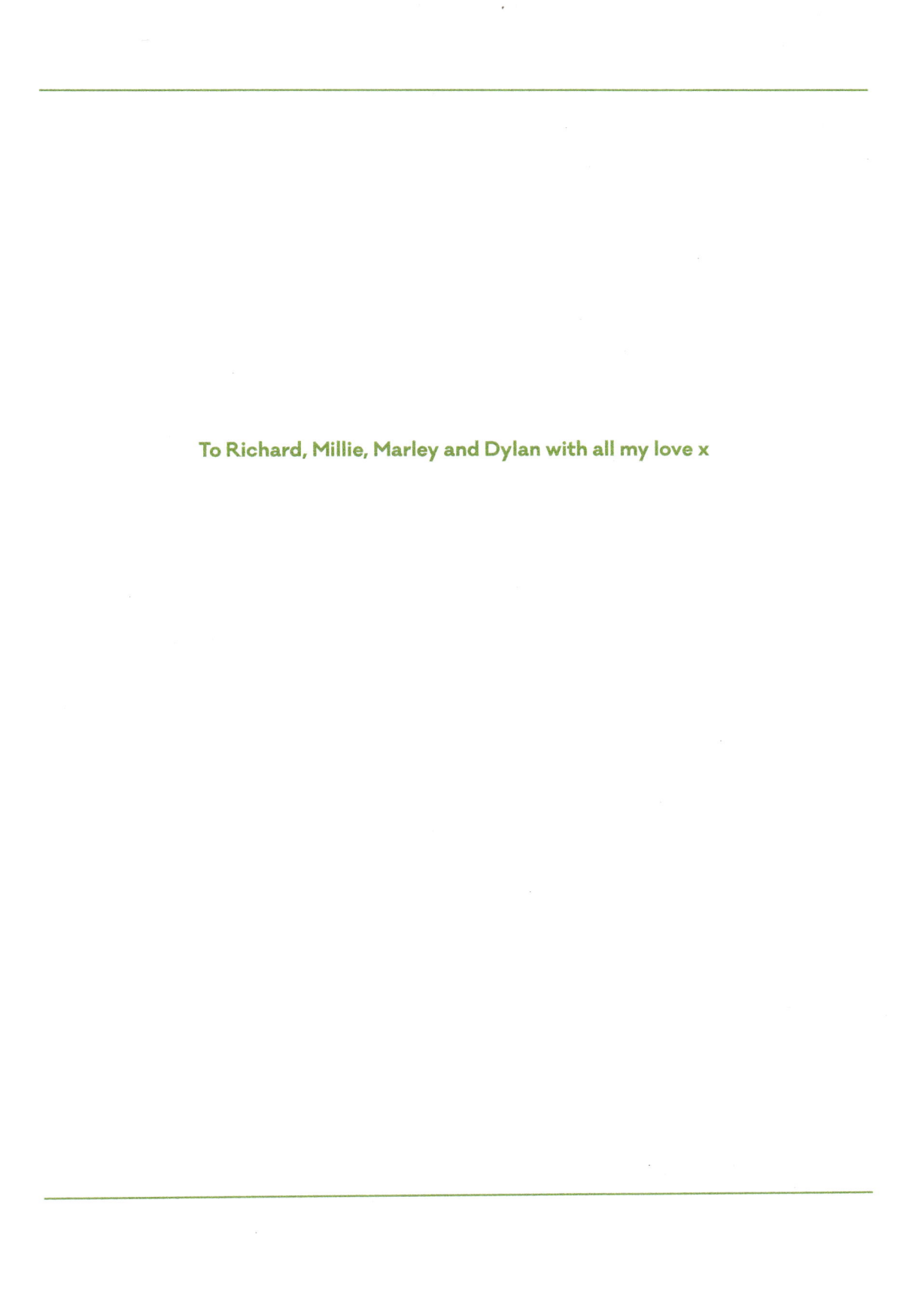

To Richard, Millie, Marley and Dylan with all my love x

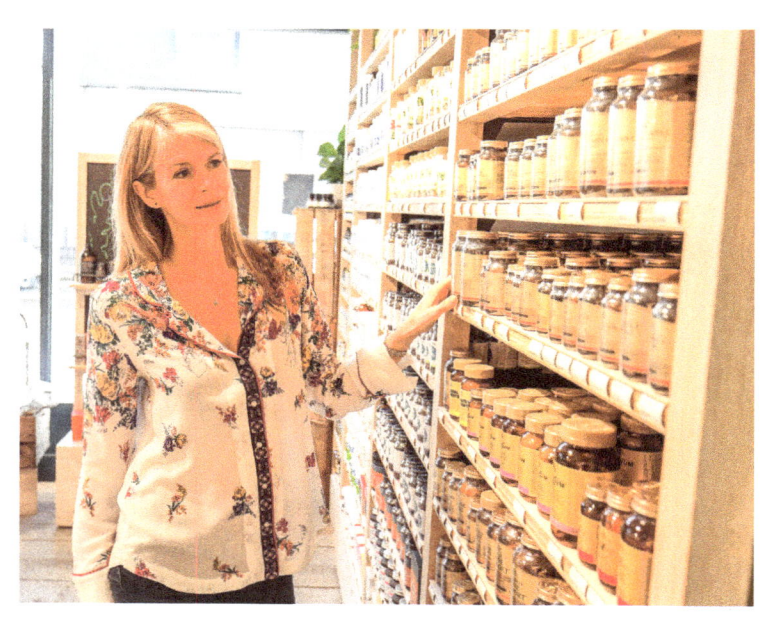

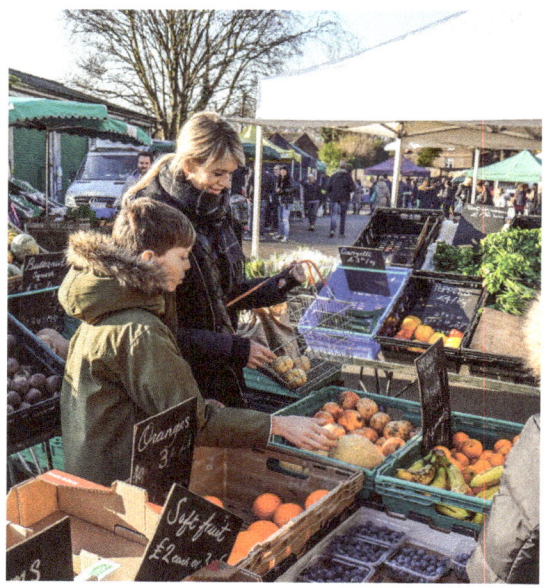

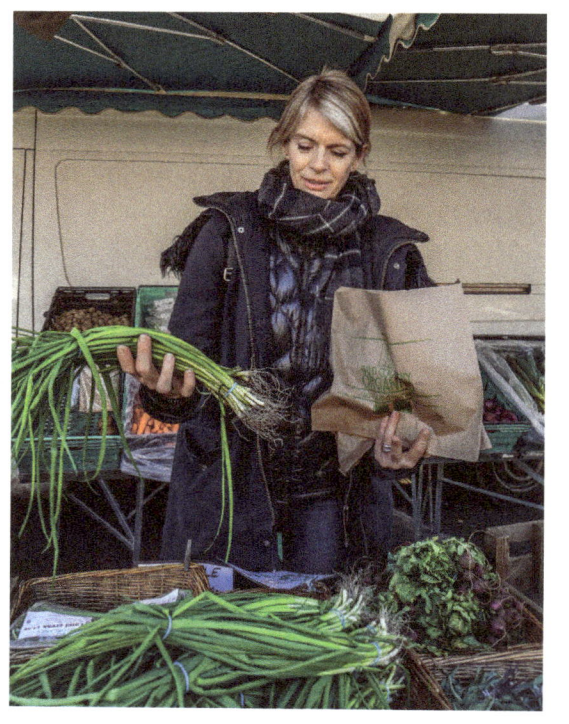

Contents

Introduction	i
Cupboard essentials	viii
Meal plans	xi
Breakfasts	1
Soups	25
Veggie sides	38
Salads	55
Mains:	67
Fishy mains	68
Meaty mains	76
Veggie mains	86
Sweet things	95
Index	109

Introduction

I wrote my first book Feed Your Health in 2010, back then I simply wanted to put together a collection of my favourite tried and tested recipes for friends and clients and was pleasantly surprised at how well it was received and by the fact that it sold out! People still come up to me and tell me what they are cooking from my Feed Your Health book and are always asking when the next book is coming out.

So here it is, I have finally produced it - a new collection of recipes! I have included a few of the old recipes from my first book in case you missed out but the vast majority of these recipes are my new personal favourites. All of these recipes are healthy, simple and delicious and have been cooked time and time again for my family, for friends and at the Cookery Workshops that I still hold regularly in my kitchen in Chiswick, West London.

This time round I didn't nag my photographer husband Richard to take the photos but used my iphone - so much easier – no hanging around and no arguments over whether to put a fork in the shot! I try to remember to instagram all of my recipes and will blog the recipe if asked, so please follow me on instagram: alligodbold.

My family are quite harsh critics - almost too honest about my food – I know if I get the thumbs up from them that a recipe can feature at a Workshop. Millie loves all things Asian, as well as being the biggest fan of harissa, avocados and goat's cheese, Marley loves meat, curries and tagines, my youngest Dylan loves fish, especially sushi and Richard loves pretty much all food - which is just as well! I think it is really important for children to try at least something of what is on the adult's plate – I rarely cook Dylan something separate as I want him to grow up experiencing all sorts of tastes and different foods, if the recipe is too spicy I might make his a little milder but I mostly resist giving him the fish finger option which I know he would sometimes prefer!

The recipes in this book are gluten free - I have learnt to cook this way as my own health is better for it but you should feel free to tweak as necessary if you prefer to cook with wheat flour or if you like to use pasta or noodles made from wheat etc. If you are in good health and have no issues digesting gluten then there is no reason to remove it, although I often tell my clients that it is worth seeing how your body reacts to a gluten free trial for a couple of weeks – if you feel much better then it is actually easier than you think to adapt to a gluten free diet.

I have been practising as a Nutritional Therapist since I graduated from London's Institute of Optimum Nutrition, way back in 1996, and what I have learnt over the last 20 years is that people really appreciate some practical cooking ideas; the majority of us are not able to follow extreme diets and want to be able to include treats and to be able to cook simple meals for family and friends. We don't want to spend hours in the kitchen so all of my recipes are simple and most of them ready to eat within 30 minutes.

I have arranged this book into sections: Breakfasts, Soups, Salads, Veggie sides, Mains and Sweet treats – so there is something for everyone and for every occasion.

I have also formulated some weekly meal plans – these plans are designed to help you if you are cleaning up your diet (detox), wanting to lose weight (weight loss), wanting to improve your digestion (gut boost), trying to beat fatigue (energy boost), or trying to sort out your mood (mood boost). There is also a vegan plan for each of these weeks. Obviously a week is not long enough to solve most health problems and if you are suffering I strongly advise you to consult a doctor or qualified nutritional therapist (www.bant.org.uk) but please let me know how you get on with these weekly plans: info@feedyourhealth.co.uk

* if the suggestions in the meal plans have an asterisk it means that the recipe is in this book

Cupboard essentials

These are very similar to those in my original book with a few important additions such as chipotle chilli paste which I honestly couldn't live without.

Once you build up these ingredients (as and when you make each recipe) it will only be a matter of time before you just need to buy fresh foods to create each recipe – you will need a large cupboard!

Oil and vinegar etc
extra virgin olive oil
extra virgin cold pressed coconut oil
cold pressed sesame oil
sea salt
black pepper
sherry vinegar
red wine vinegar
white wine vinegar
apple cider vinegar ('with the mother')

Marigold bouillon – reduced salt
Marigold Engevita nutritional yeast flakes
wholegrain mustard
Dijon mustard
tahini

Asian flavours
Clearspring mirin
Clearspring brown rice vinegar
Clearspring tamari soy sauce
Clearspring sushi ginger
Thai fish sauce
Thai red curry paste (Thai Taste)
Clearspring sweet white miso paste
nori seaweed sheets
Vietnamese rice wrappers

Herbs and spices
nigella seeds
mustard seeds
cloves
curry powder
cayenne pepper
chilli flakes
caraway seeds
cardamom pods
Za'atar
garam masala
turmeric
ground cumin seeds
whole cumin seeds
ground coriander seeds
whole coriander seeds
smoked paprika (Brindisa La Chinata)
paprika
bayleaves
kaffir lime leaves
mixed herbs
oregano
chipotle chilli paste
tamarind paste
Beluza rose harissa

Gluten free grains
Nairns gf oatcakes
brown basmati rice
quinoa
100% buckwheat noodles
Thai flat rice noodles
gluten free oats
brown rice flour (Infinity Foods)
Doves Farm gf brown bread flour
buckwheat flour
coconut flour

Baking
fast acting yeast
gluten free baking powder
nuts – brazils, walnuts, cashews, hazelnuts, almonds, pistachios (unsalted & unroasted)
ground almonds
seeds – sesame, sunflower, pumpkin, chia
Linwoods ground flax seeds
psyllium husks
vanilla bean extract (Nielson Massey)
cacoa powder
ground cinnamon
100% maple syrup/date syrup/organic honey
Organic dates, figs, apricots and raisins

More essentials
capers
chickpeas, canned
tomatoes, canned
beans – cannellini, borlotti, haricot, black, canned
tomato puree
passata
red lentils
Puy lentils
sardines, canned
chargrilled peppers in a jar
coconut milk, canned

For breakfast
Plenish almond milk/
Koko coconut milk
maca, lacuma & acai berry powder
unsweetened peanut butter
almond butter

Fresh essentials
onion, garlic, chillies, ginger
lemons, limes

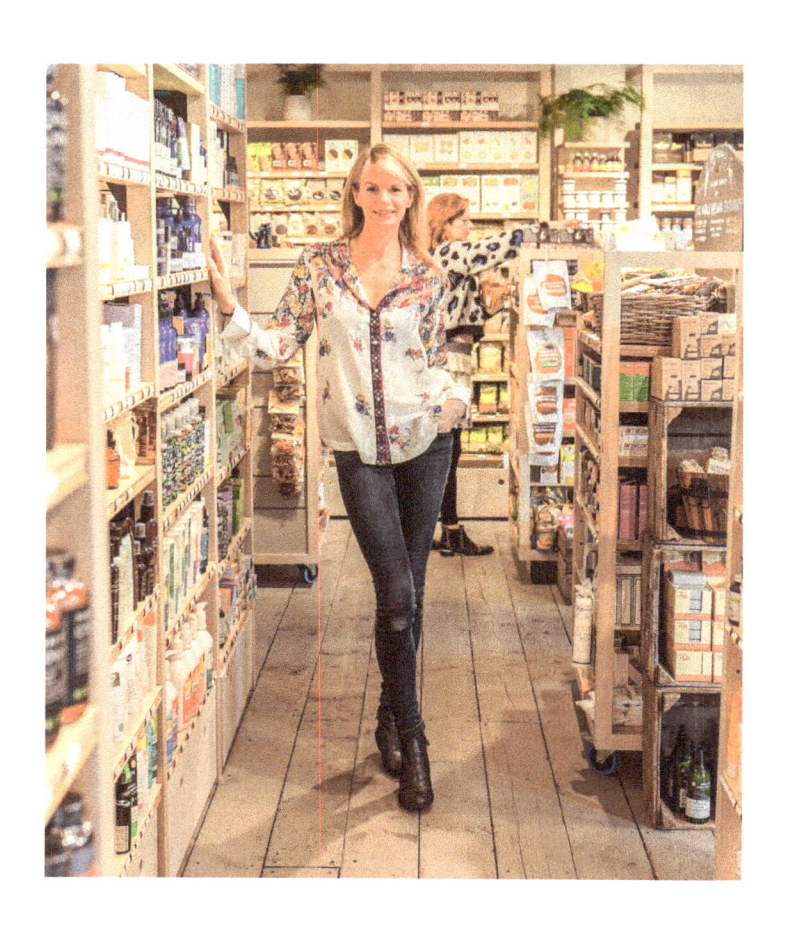

Meal plans

Detox

This is the meal plan for you if you have been overdoing it – a boozy Christmas or a Summer of Rosé wine or perhaps just too many coffees and teas or too many take-aways.

Detoxification takes place in the body all the time; the liver, skin, lungs, kidneys and gut all play a part. This week's diet is designed to particularly support the liver as it rids your body of stored toxins, for some people this might result in headaches, tiredness and even aches and pains, for others there are no outward signs that anything is happening, it all depends on the state of your health and how you have been treating your body. This week you should try and take it easy, avoid strenuous exercise and drink plenty of water.

Start each day with a mug of hot water and lemon – cut a slice of lemon and pour on some freshly boiled water - this is a great start to the day and gives your liver a break from processing the caffeine in your normal tea or coffee.

The snack each day is a green juice – you can use whatever green vegetables you have to hand but cruciferous vegetables such as kale, cabbage and broccoli are really good liver boosting greens. Add a large handful of greens to a powerful blender with some ice, cold water and half an apple, pear or a slice of pineapple for sweetness, whizz into a refreshing juice, adding more water to thin so that the juice is not too soupy. You could add a dessertspoon of ground flaxseeds to boost detox via the gut.

Don't go hungry, if you need more food then add some Nutty Seed Bread, Flax Seed Crackers or some gluten free oatcakes – all of these are great spread with almond butter or hummus if you need something between meals or to accompany lunch.

Detox Meal Plan - Meat and Fish

	Breakfast	**Lunch**	**Dinner**
1	Hot lemon water *Herb omelette	*Pomegranate, chickpea and mint salad	*Chimi-churri chicken with *Sweet potato wedges and steamed broccoli
2	Hot lemon water Green smoothie	*Bissara broadbean soup	*Fish and salsa parcels with *Cauliflower rice
3	Hot lemon water Poached eggs with avocado on *Nutty seed bread	*Butternut squash, kale & feta salad	*Coconut & chickpea curry
4	Hot lemon water *Muesli with berries and nut milk	*Lentil, tomato & spinach soup	*Turkey koftas with tahini dressing and brown basmati rice
5	Hot lemon water Boiled eggs with *Flax seed crackers	*Avocado, tomato & coriander salad	*Cauliflower pizza
6	Hot lemon water *Nutty granola and berries	*Moroccan beetroot dip with mixed salad	*Mexican salmon with guacamole and brown basmati rice
7	Hot lemon water *Scrambled eggs with smoked salmon	*Roasted pepper soup	Roast lamb with roasted beetroot, squash & garlic and steamed broccoli

Detox Meal Plan - vegan

	Breakfast	Lunch	Dinner
1	Hot lemon water *Chai yoghurt pot	*Pomegranate, chickpea and mint salad	*Tofu Pad Prik curry with basmati brown rice
2	Hot lemon water *Berry smoothie	*Bissara broadbean soup with *Flax seed crackers	*White Beanotto with mushroom and spinach
3	Hot lemon water *Nutty granola	*Butternut squash and kale salad	*Cauliflower pizza
4	Hot lemon water *Muesli, berries and nut milk	*Lentil, tomato & spinach soup	*Ratatouille with puy lentils
5	Hot lemon water *Smoothie bowl	*Avocado, tomato & coriander salad	*Coconut & chickpea curry
6	Hot lemon water Mushrooms, tomatoes and spinach with toasted gluten free bread	*Moroccan beetroot dip with mixed salad	*Quinoa burgers with *Winter slaw
7	Hot lemon water *Buckwheat pancakes with coconut yoghurt	*Roasted pepper soup	*Gado Gado vegetables with satay sauce

Weight Loss

The weight loss meal plan introduces the concept of reducing your intake of starchy carbs. It avoids all processed and refined foods and is free from added sugar. Carbs all eventually break down into sugars, which can contribute to weight gain, so this week's plan allows starchy carbs at breakfast and lunch but restricts them in the evening.

It is advisable to eat every 4 hours – if you have to wait longer than that between lunch and dinner then snack on a few raw nuts, a green juice or a slice of Nutty Seed bread spread with a teaspoon of nut butter.

There is protein at every meal, plenty of good fats and fibre to stabilize blood sugar levels - good blood sugar balance is key to weight loss.

Weight Loss Meal Plan - Meat and Fish

	Breakfast	Lunch	Dinner
1	Hot lemon water / green tea *Green smoothie bowl	Cold roast meat with mixed salad	*Carrot bolognaise with courgette spaghetti
2	Hot lemon water / green tea *Nutty granola with yoghurt and berries	*Japanese salad with tofu	*Quick lemon chicken with asparagus and green beans
3	Hot lemon water / green tea *Fresh herb omelette with *Nutty seed bread	*Roasted red pepper soup with *Flax seed crackers	*Japanese blackened salmon with *Ginger broccoli and pak choi
4	Hot lemon water / green tea *Berry smoothie	*Avocado & tomato salad with smoked mackerel	*Fish and salsa parcels with steamed vegetables
5	Hot lemon water / green tea Poached eggs & spinach on *Nutty seed bread	*Lentil and tomato soup with *Flax seed crackers	*Favourite chicken curry with cauliflower rice
6	Hot lemon water / green tea *Buckwheat pancakes with yoghurt & berries	*Courgetti with pistachio pesto and feta	*Seared sirloin steak with rocket and chicory salad
7	Hot lemon water / green tea *Grilled fig with Parma ham, Greek yoghurt & pistachios	*Roast chicken with butternut squash	*Smoked salmon paté on *Flax seed crackers with mixed salad

Weight Loss Meal Plan - vegan

	Breakfast	Lunch	Dinner
1	Hot lemon water / green tea *Green smoothie bowl	*Bissara broadbean soup	*Carrot bolognaise with courgette spaghetti
2	Hot lemon water / green tea *Nutty granola with coconut yoghurt and berries	*Japanese salad with tofu	*Coconut & chickpea curry with *Cauliflower rice
3	Hot lemon water / green tea *Chai yoghurt pot with berries	*Roasted red pepper soup with *Flax seed crackers	*Roasted miso aubergine with *Ginger broccoli and pak choi
4	Hot lemon water / green tea *Berry smoothie	*Avocado and tomato salad with smoked tofu	*White beanotto with mixed salad
5	Hot lemon water / green tea *Grilled fig with pistachios and coconut yoghurt	*Lentil, spinach and tomato soup with *Flax seed crackers	*Tofu Pak Prik curry with *Cauliflower rice
6	Hot lemon water / green tea *Buckwheat pancakes with coconut yoghurt & berries	*Courgetti with pistachio pesto	*Cauliflower pizza
7	Hot lemon water / green tea *Home made baked beans with wilted spinach on *Nutty seed bread	*Quinoa burgers with tahini dressing and salsa	*Fresh spring rolls

Gut Boost

Start each day with a mug of hot water and lemon – cut a slice of lemon and pour on some freshly boiled water – this helps to stimulate digestion preparing your body for food.

As well as being gluten free this week's diet is also dairy free – gluten and dairy are often poorly tolerated and worth taking a break from to see how your digestive system responds. If you feel no different you can resume eating these foods at the end of the week.

Everyone is different and this diet will not work for absolutely everyone with digestive complaints. If adding fibre rich foods to your diet makes you feel worse or causes diarrhoea or constipation then you should see a qualified nutritionist or your GP as you may be better off, in the short term, on a low Fodmap diet – this is a diet which restricts highly fermentable carbohydrates including onions, garlic, leeks, chickpeas etc. A nutritionist might also decide to organise a test for SIBO (small intestine bowel overgrowth) which, if present, requires a special dietary approach, liver support and antimicrobials.

Some people experiencing digestive symptoms might have a food sensitivity to something they are eating, others may be low in stomach acid or digestive enzymes. If you follow this diet and still experience problems then please consult a doctor/nutritionist as they will help to resolve any other issues.

This week you should snack only if you are truly hungry, avoid grazing on food in order to give your digestive system a well deserved rest between meals. Aim for 4 hour spacing between meals. Suitable snacks if you really are hungry might be a couple of oatcakes with some nut butter, a small handful of raw nuts or some coconut yoghurt with added berries and seeds. Aim to leave a minimum of 12 hours between finishing dinner and breakfast the next morning.

Gut Boost Meal Plan - Meat and Fish

	Breakfast	Lunch	Dinner
1	Hot lemon water *Scrambled egg with smoked salmon and *Nutty seed bread	Salad with *Sauerkraut *Sprouted seeds, avocado and *Tempeh	*Chicken soup using chicken stock and vegetables
2	Hot lemon water *Stewed apple with coconut yoghurt, chia seeds and berries	Sardines mashed with sherry vinegar, salad vegetables and *Flax seed crackers	*Miso salmon with asparagus and *sweet potato wedges
3	Hot lemon water Mushroom & spinach omelette	*Apple, almond & rocket salad with apple cider vinegar dressing and a bowl of *Chicken soup	*Favourite chicken curry with coconut yoghurt and brown basmati rice
4	Hot lemon water *Bircher museli with nut milk, berries and ground flax seeds	*Roasted red pepper soup with gluten free oatcakes	*Chickpea & kale hotpot
5	Hot lemon water Boiled eggs with *Nutty seed bread	Salad with smoked salmon and *Sprouted seeds with *Flax seed crackers	*veggie bolognaise with courgette spaghetti
6	Hot lemon water *Nutty granola with coconut yoghurt	*Lentil, spinach and tomato soup	Seafood sushi
7	Hot lemon water Poached eggs with smashed avocado on *Nutty seed bread	*Smoked mackerel paté with salad and *Sprouted seeds	Roast chicken with *Roasted vegetables and greens

Gut Boost Meal Plan - vegan

	Breakfast	**Lunch**	**Dinner**
1	Hot lemon water *Nutty seed bread with nut butter and berries	Salad with *Sauerkraut *Sprouted seeds, avocado and *Tempeh	*Tofu Pad Prik with basmati brown rice
2	Hot lemon water *Stewed apple with coconut yoghurt, chia seeds and berries	Minestrone soup with *Flax seed crackers	*Quinoa burgers with tahini dressing and tomato salsa
3	Hot lemon water *Nutty granola with coconut yoghurt and berries	*Pomegranate, chickpea & mint salad	*White beanotto with spinach
4	Hot lemon water *Bircher museli with nut milk, berries and ground flax seeds	*Cashew cream cheese on gluten free bread with salad	*Chickpea & kale hotpot
5	Hot lemon water Smashed avocado on *Nutty seed bread	*Minestrone soup with *Flax seed crackers	*Sticky, spicy aubergine with large salad and hummous
6	Hot lemon water Mushrooms and tomatoes with spinach with *Nutty seed bread	*Fresh spring rolls	*Thai Tofu Laksa with brown basmati rice
7	Hot lemon water *Buckwheat pancakes with coconut yoghurt and berries	*Home made baked beans with wilted spinach on *Nutty seed bread	*Roasted vegetables and greens

Energy Boost

Balancing blood sugar levels is essential if you are struggling with low energy or if you suffer from sugar cravings. Eating in a way that causes sugars to be released into the blood very slowly is key for maintaining a good level of energy, as well as preventing the development of diabetes and can be very helpful for weight loss.

This week's plan contains practically no added sugar and focuses on including a good source of protein at every meal. Protein starts its digestion in the stomach, which means that the carbs eaten alongside it are held in the stomach for longer before they reach the intestines where they can be broken down into sugars.

Fibre is also important for slowing down the release of sugars from carbs, so this week's recipes contain plenty of fibrous vegetables. Grains are kept to a minimum as even whole grains are ultimately a concentrated source of sugars and can upset blood sugar levels in some people.

If hungry opt for a handful of raw nuts or try some vegetable crudities dipped in almond butter. If you are desperately craving something sweet try a Maca Smoothie. You could also try a mug of Peppermint and Liquorice tea, as this often satisfies a sweet craving.

SNACKS: The idea is to stay fuelled but to avoid constant snacking by eating enough at meal times - add crackers with nut butter if you need more at lunch times or as a snack during the day, or choose a piece of fruit with some raw nuts.

Energy Boost Meal Plan - Meat and Fish

	Breakfast	Lunch	Dinner
1	Hot lemon water / green tea 2 boiled eggs with a slice of *Nutty seed bread or flax seed crackers	*Lentil, tomato and spinach soup	*Chicken chimichurri with asparagus and puy lentils
2	Hot lemon water / green tea *Yoghurt berry smoothie with walnuts and cinnamon	Smoked salmon with *Avocado & tomato salad	*Mexican bean soup with salsa
3	Hot lemon water / green tea 2 poached eggs with grilled tomatoes, *Nutty seed bread or *Flax seed crackers	Seafood sushi	*Miso salmon with radish and courgette salad
4	Hot lemon water / green tea *Smashed avocado with chilli & lime on *Nutty seed bread or *Flax seed crackers	*Roasted butternut squash soup	*Turkey koftas with *Tahini dressing
5	Hot lemon water / green tea Yoghurt with rolled oats, berries and cinnamon	Chicken salad with romaine lettuce and apple cider vinaigrette	*Tofu Pad Prik curry with *Cauliflower rice
6	Hot lemon water / green tea Hard boiled eggs with hummus on *Nutty seed bread or *Flax seed crackers	*Tom Yum soup	*Moroccan fish tagine with new potatoes
7	Hot lemon water / green tea *Scrambled eggs and smoked salmon with *Nutty seed bread or *Flax seed crackers	*Smoked mackerel paté with *Flax seed crackers and salad	*Grilled lamb with herby salsa verde and roasted butternut squash

Energy Boost Meal Plan - vegan

	Breakfast	**Lunch**	**Dinner**
1	Hot lemon water / green tea *Nutty seed bread or *Flax seed crackers with nut butter or avocado	*Lentil, tomato and spinach soup	*Chickpea curry with brown basmati rice
2	Hot lemon water / green tea *Coconut yoghurt berry smoothie with walnuts and cinnamon	*Japanese salad with smoked tofu	*Mexican bean soup with salsa
3	Hot lemon water / green tea Grilled tomatoes on *Nutty seed bread or *Flax seed crackers	*Fresh spring rolls	*Quinoa burgers with *Tahini dressing and tomato salsa
4	Hot lemon water / green tea *Smashed avocado with chilli & lime on *Nutty seed bread or *Flax seed crackers	*Roasted butternut squash soup	*Tofu Pad Prik curry with *Cauliflower rice
5	Hot lemon water / green tea Coconut yoghurt with rolled oats, berries and cinnamon	*Pomegranate, chickpea & mint salad	*White beanotto with spinach
6	Hot lemon water / green tea *Almond pancakes with sautéed mushrooms and tomatoes	*Tom Yum soup	*Thai tofu laksa
7	Hot lemon water / green tea *Scrambled tofu with *Nutty seed bread or *Flax seed crackers	*Cashew cheese with *Flax seed crackers and salad	*Gado Gado

Mood Boost

Our mood may be affected by blood sugar swings as glucose is the primary fuel source for the brain, so it is essential to keep blood sugar levels stable – eat regularly, try to include protein at every meal and avoid processed foods. The neurotransmitters, which are chemicals in the body that control our mood, are made from proteins and are therefore dependant on a good intake of protein. Neurotransmitters require lots of nutrients to act as cofactors for their formation; nutrients such as magnesium, zinc and iron are all important.

Serotonin is the neurotransmitter that helps us to feel relaxed and is made from the amino acid tryptophan – this is rich in many foods such as eggs, soy, spirulina, fish, seeds, pulses and meat. Tryptophan requires insulin to get it into the blood stream. Insulin needs to be released steadily, rather than in massive spikes, and this is best achieved by eating a diet rich in protein, with some slow release carbs and good fats.

B vitamins and magnesium are particularly important for controlling stress. Good sources of B vitamins are liver, chicken, eggs, dairy and green leafy vegetables. Magnesium is rich in nuts and seeds, green vegetables and pulses.

Essential fats from oily fish, nuts and seeds and their oils, are important for mood and good cognition.

Green tea is recommended, as in all the meal plans, for its antioxidant properties. Green tea is also a good source of l-theanine which is important for reducing anxiety.

Mood Boost Meal Plan - Meat and Fish

	Breakfast	Lunch	Dinner
1	Green tea *Almond and seedy granola with fresh berries	*Butternut squash, kale and feta salad	*Sticky & spicy aubergine with brown basmati rice
2	Green tea Poached eggs and mashed avocado on *Nutty seed bread	*Lentil and spinach soup	*Miso salmon with courgette & radish salad
3	Green tea * Yoghurt smoothie with berries and seeds	*Chickpea and feta salad	*Chicken chimichurri with *Cauliflower rice and green beans
4	Green tea *Spinach omelette	*Minestrone soup with *Nutty seed bread or *Flax seed crackers	*Courgetti with pistachio pesto and feta
5	Green tea *Porridge with berries and maple syrup	*Salmon paté and salad with *Flax seed crackers	*Minute steak with chicory & rocket salad and sweet potato wedges
6	Green tea *Ham & egg frittatas	*Fresh spring rolls with prawns and avocado	*Salmon burgers with fruity salsa
7	Green tea *Scrambled eggs and smoked salmon on *Nutty seed bread	*Pear and fennel soup	*Roast chicken with butternut squash and green vegetables

Mood Boost Meal Plan - vegan

	Breakfast	Lunch	Dinner
1	Green tea *Almond and seedy granola with fresh berries	*Butternut squash, kale and *Tempeh salad	*Roasted harissa aubergine with green beans and *Cauliflower rice
2	Green tea *Smashed avocado on *Nutty seed bread	*Lentil and spinach soup	*Japanese salad with stir fried tofu
3	Green tea *Coconut yoghurt smoothie	*Chickpea salad	*Beanotto with spinach and mushrooms
4	Green tea *Scrambled tofu and *Flax seed crackers	*Minestrone soup with *Nutty seed bread or *Flax seed crackers	*Courgetti with pistachio pesto and feta
5	Green tea *Porridge with berries and maple syrup	*Broad bean soup with *Flax seed crackers and salad	*Tofu Laksa with pak choi
6	Green tea *vegan buckwheat pancakes with coconut yoghurt and berries	*Fresh spring rolls with avocado and vegetables	*Quinoa burgers with tomato salsa, harissa dressing and green salad
7	Green tea *Scrambled tofu and sautéed mushrooms with *Nutty seed bread	*Pear and fennel soup	*Cauliflower pizza with artichoke, asparagus and rocket topping

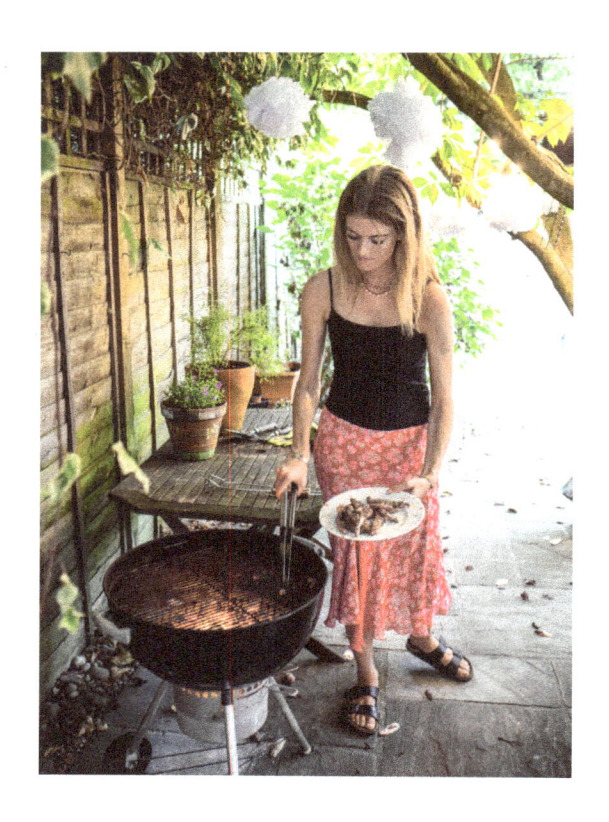

Recipes

Breakfast

Avoid eating as soon as you get up, give your digestive system a chance to wake up – try starting the day with a cup of hot water poured onto a slice of lemon to get the digestive juices flowing.

It's a good idea to include eggs for breakfast as they are a simple way to provide protein and fat, which will satisfy your appetite for longer than a bowl of cereal or toast.

If you don't like the idea of eggs make sure you include protein from other sources: natural yoghurt, nuts and seeds, nut and seed butters or smoked salmon are all good choices.

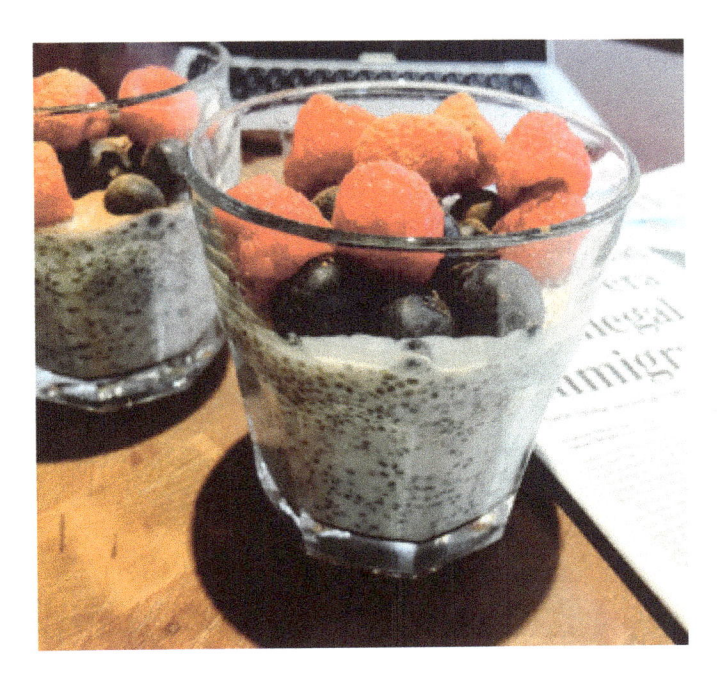

Scrambled eggs, smoked salmon and chives

Serves 1

2 eggs
1 slice of smoked salmon, cut into ribbons
a few chives, chopped finely and/or dill
1 tsp butter/coconut oil

Whisk the eggs while you melt the butter/oil in a heavy based pan. Add eggs to a pan and stir gently with a wooden spoon.

Add the salmon and herbs and serve immediately. Serve with a couple of Seedy Crackers or a slice of good quality gluten free toast.

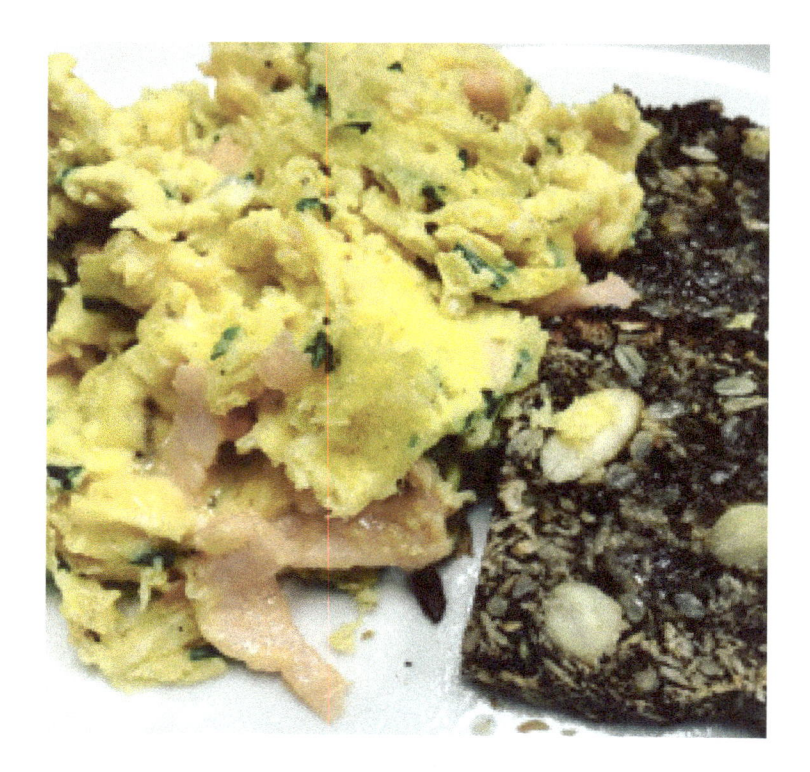

Spinach omelette

Serves 1

2 eggs, beaten
large handful spinach
1 tsp coconut oil or butter

Melt the oil/butter in a large heavy based pan. Pour the eggs into the pan and swirl around so that the eggs cover the entire base of the pan.

When the bottom of the omelette is cooked spread the spinach over the omelette.

Using a palette knife gently roll the omelette from the edge of the pan to make a 'roll'.

To make a herb omelette substitute spinach for herbs of your choice.

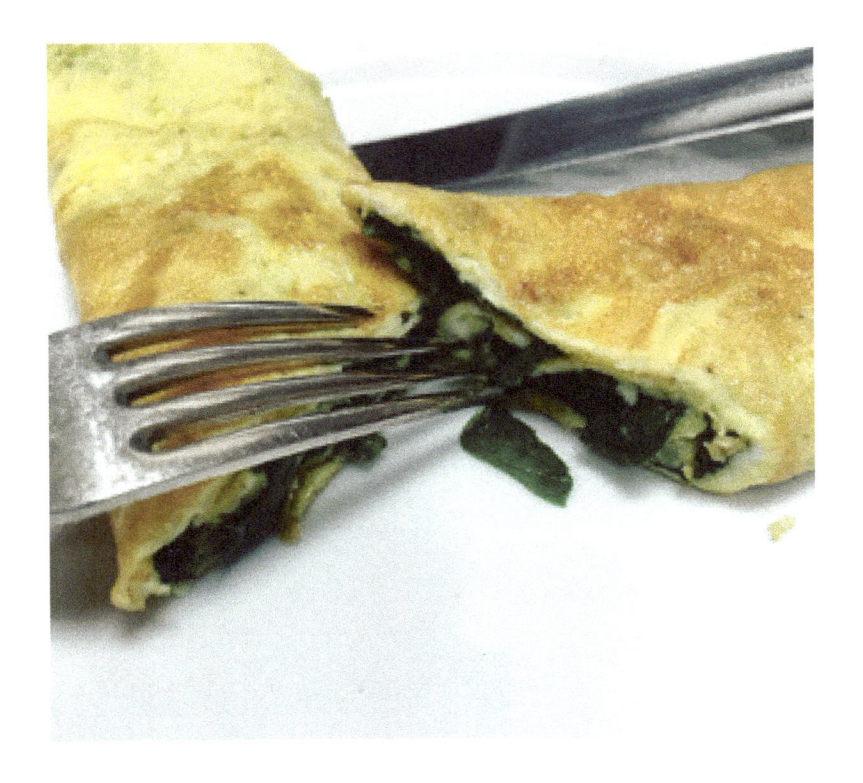

Mini ham and egg frittatas

Serves 2-3

coconut oil for greasing
6 slices Parma ham
4 eggs

black pepper
2 spring onions, finely chopped

Preheat the oven to 200°C.

Lightly grease a 6 hole muffin tin with coconut oil or butter.

Place a slice of ham in each hole and shape it to form a cup. Beat the eggs in a bowl, season with black pepper and stir in the spring onion.

Pour the egg mix into the ham cups and bake in the oven for about 15 mins until the eggs have set.

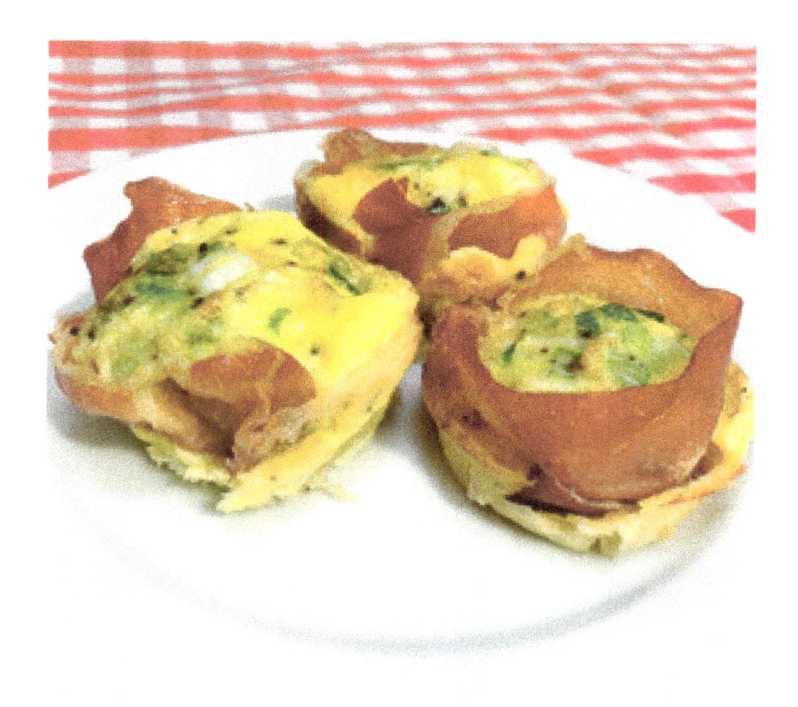

Berber eggs

Serves 2

1 red onion, finely chopped
half red chilli, finely chopped
2 garlic cloves, crushed
400g can chopped tomatoes

150g cherry tomatoes, halved
half tsp smoked paprika
4 eggs
2 tbsp fresh coriander

Heat the frying pan and in a little oil sauté the onion, chilli and garlic for a few minutes. Add the chopped tomatoes, paprika and a little water and cook for 5 mins.

Crack the eggs into the sauce, cover the pan with a lid and cook for approx. 8 mins. until the egg whites are set. Scatter with coriander and serve immediately.

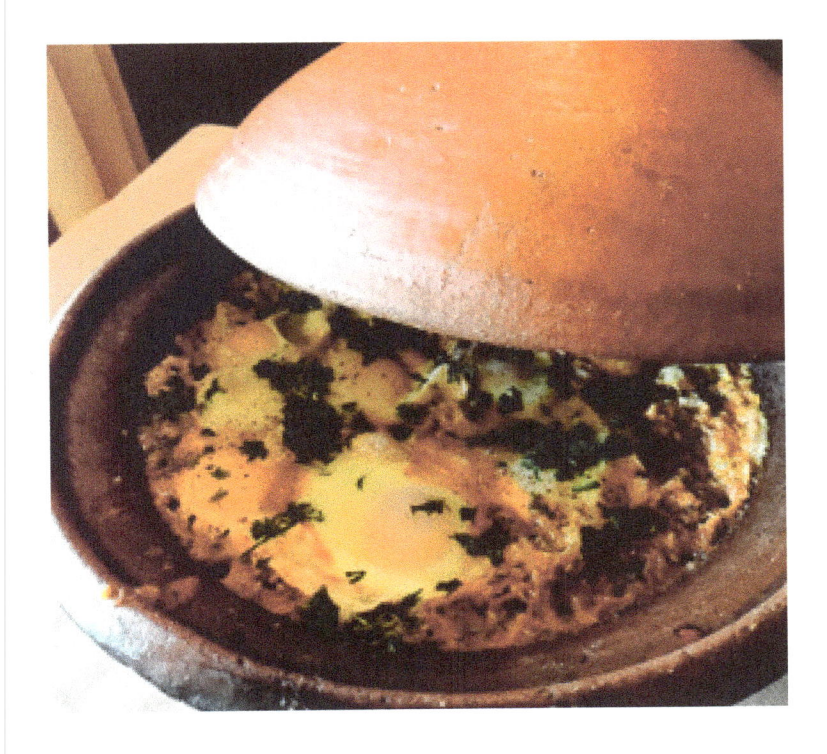

Scrambled tofu

Serves 2

1 tsp nutritional yeast flakes
1/4 tsp turmeric
1/4 tsp ground cumin
1/4 tsp paprika
1 tbsp water
pinch sea salt

black pepper
olive oil
1 spring onion, finely diced
1 clove garlic, finely chopped
1/2 package firm tofu, very well drained
1 tbsp parsley, finely chopped

In a small bowl, mix together nutritional yeast, turmeric, cumin, paprika, water, salt, and pepper. Set aside.

Heat a little olive oil in a frying pan. Once hot, add spring onion and garlic and sauté until fragrant, about 2 minutes. Crumble tofu into the pan, breaking it up with your fingers. Pour seasoning over tofu and mix well, trying to colour as much tofu as possible.

Cook for 2 minutes or until tofu is hot throughout. Toss in parsley and continue to stir for another 1 to 2 minutes.

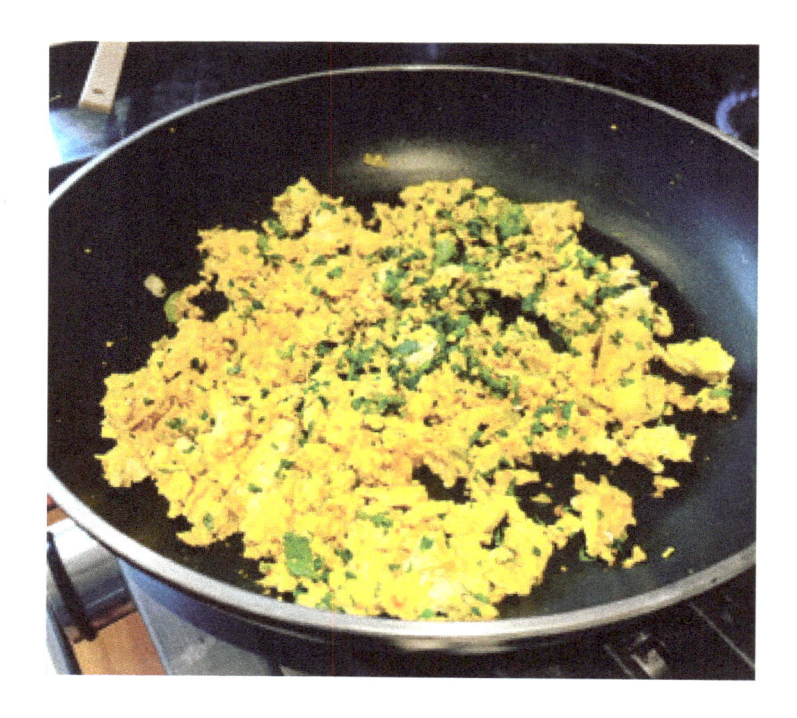

Yoghurt add-ins

Natural yoghurt makes a great base for a healthy breakfast. You can jazz it up with any of the following ingredients:

1 tbsp of oats
1 dessertspoon mixed seeds
(eg: sesame, pumpkin, sunflower, flax, poppy, hemp, chia) or mixed raw nuts
a handful of berries
fresh fruit slices or stewed apple
1 tsp bee pollen
1 tsp maca powder
1 tsp lacuma powder

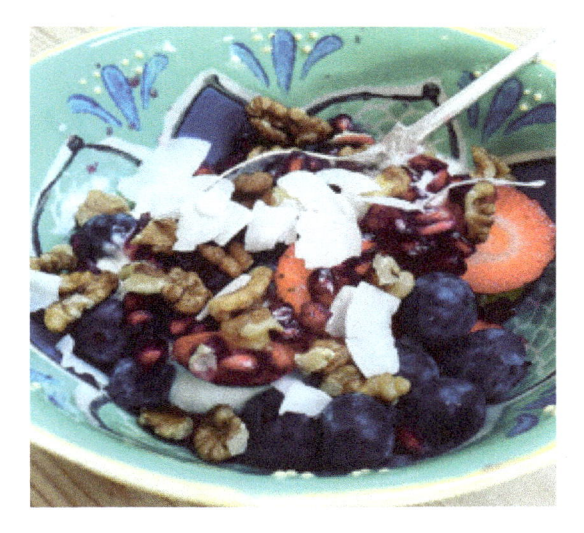

Stewed apple

Stewed apple helps to heal the gut and is a good food to include regularly if you are struggling with digestive or autoimmune issues.

Serves 4

3 Bramley apples
maple syrup
1 tsp ground cinnamon

Peel and core the apples and cut into bite-size chunks. Put the apple in a saucepan with just a splash of water to cover the bottom of the pan, a drizzle of maple syrup and a teaspoon of ground cinnamon.

Cook with a lid on for about 5-7 minutes so that the apple stays in chunks, leave it much longer and you will have apple sauce!

Chia yoghurt pots

Chia seeds expand in liquid and, along with the coconut yoghurt, are very filling so this breakfast keeps you feeling full for longer.

Serves 2

250g coconut yoghurt
125ml Koko coconut milk
40g chia seeds
1 tsp vanilla extract (Nielsen Massey)

1 tbsp honey or maple syrup
handful of blueberries and raspberries
ground cinnamon

Mix the yoghurt, coconut milk, chia seeds, vanilla extract and honey/syrup in a bowl. Leave in fridge for at least an hour or overnight so that the chia seeds become soft and gelatinous.

Divide the chia mixture between 2 glass tumblers or jars and top with fresh berries sprinkled with a pinch of cinnamon.

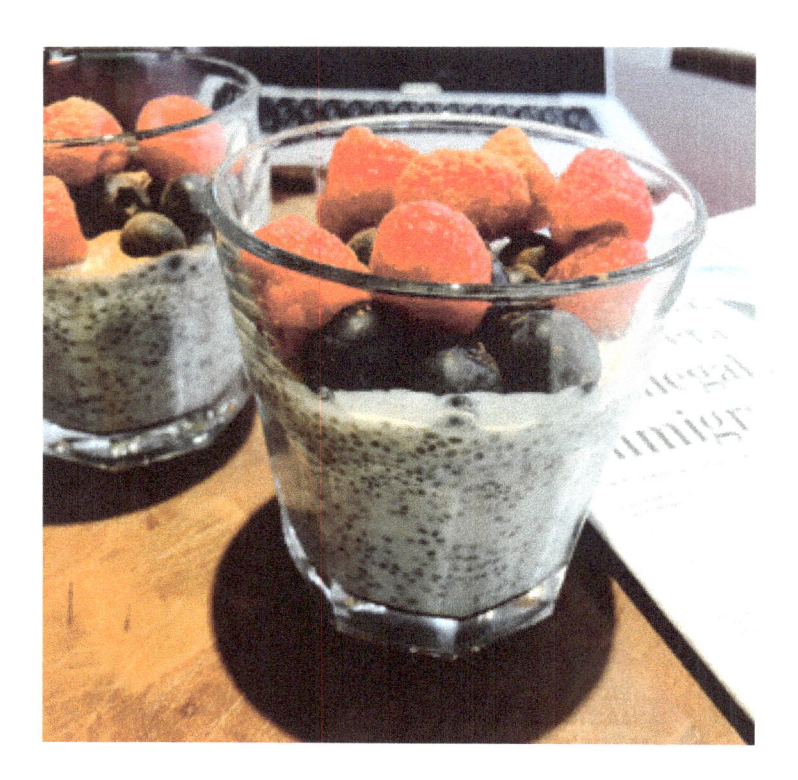

Grilled figs

Serves 1

2 small figs
100 ml Greek yoghurt
1 tbsp shelled pistachios (raw, unsalted) crushed

Cut figs in half and grill seed side up until golden. Spoon over yoghurt and sprinkle with pistachios.

You may like to serve this with sliced avocado and a slice of Parma ham.

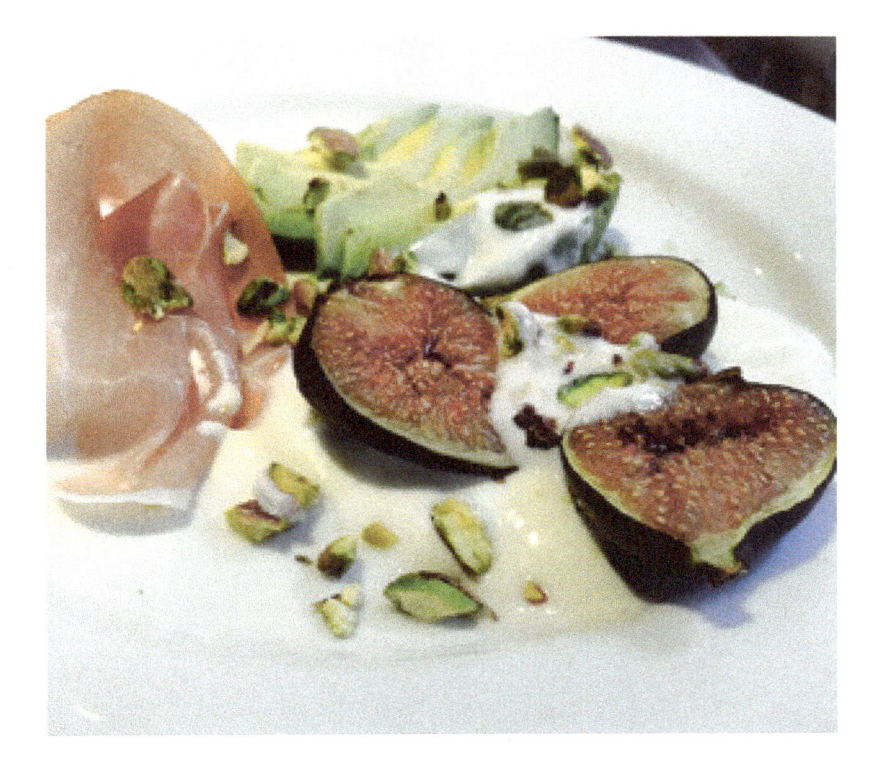

Smoothies

'Smoothie bowls' are definitely a thing – the idea is to have a go at adding interesting toppings which look great on Instagram! If you have the time and the inclination then here are a couple of smoothie bowl ideas.

Green smoothie bowl

Serves 2

1 frozen banana
half a ripe avocado
handful of spinach or kale
250ml soya, coconut or almond milk (unsweetened)

Put the banana, avocado, greens and milk plus any of your favourite add-ins (see list for yoghurt) in a blender and blend on high speed until completely smooth.

Pour the smoothie into a bowl and top with anything you like – fresh fruit slices, berries, desiccated coconut, a swirl of nut butter etc.
– you can be as inventive as you like.

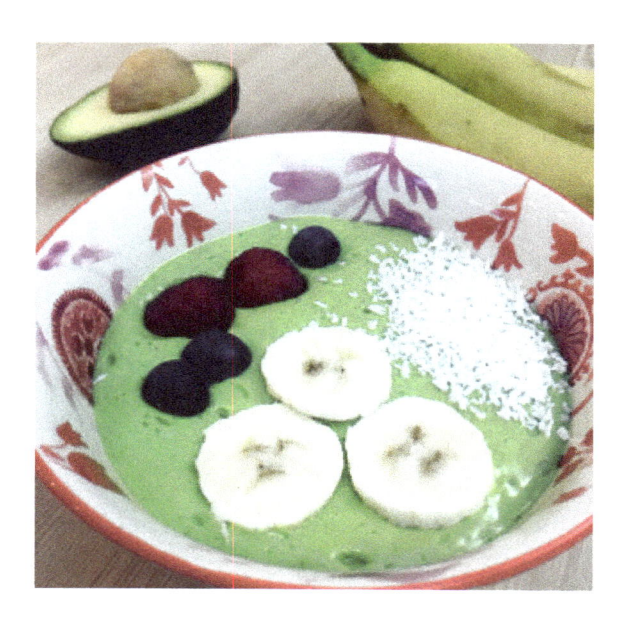

Pink smoothie bowl

Serves 1

50g frozen berries
100ml soya, coconut or almond milk
1 frozen banana
1 dessert spoon of acai berry powder

Follow the same method as for the Green Smoothie bowl, adding your favourite add-ins and toppings.

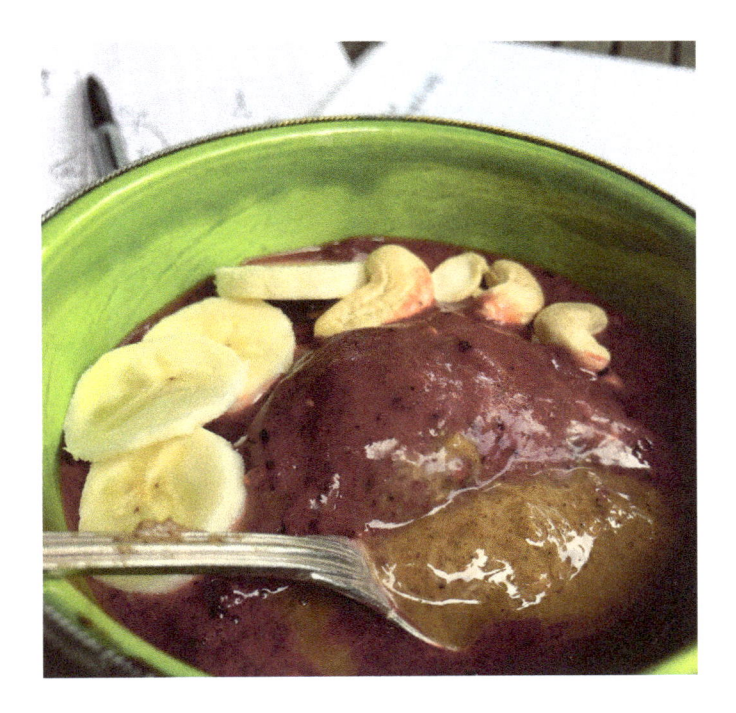

Yoghurt berry smoothie with walnuts and cinnamon

Serves 1

100g frozen berries
100g natural yoghurt (dairy/soya/coconut.. – your choice)
100ml of milk (dairy/soya/almond/coconut, etc.)
25g walnuts
half a frozen banana
pinch of ground cinnamon

Combine all the ingredients in a powerful blender and blitz to a smooth consistency, adding more milk if you prefer a thinner texture.

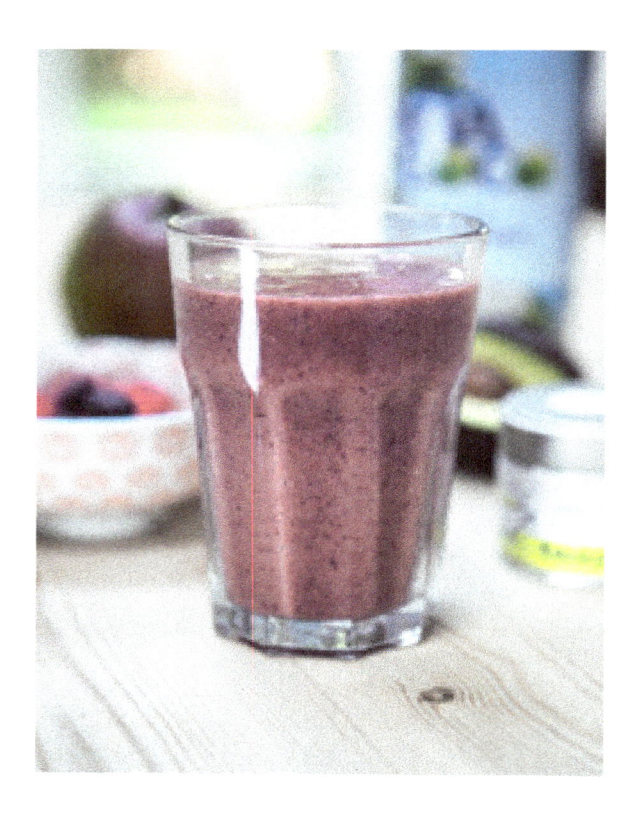

Oaty options

Granola, porridge and muesli bring variety to breakfast-time, be sure to serve with yoghurt and nuts and seeds so that you start the day with adequate protein.

Muesli

250g gluten free rolled oats
handful of dried fruit, chopped (raisins, apricots, figs)
large handful of raw nuts, chopped
100g ground flax seeds
100g mixed seeds
pinch of ground cinnamon

Combine all the ingredients and keep in an air-tight container.

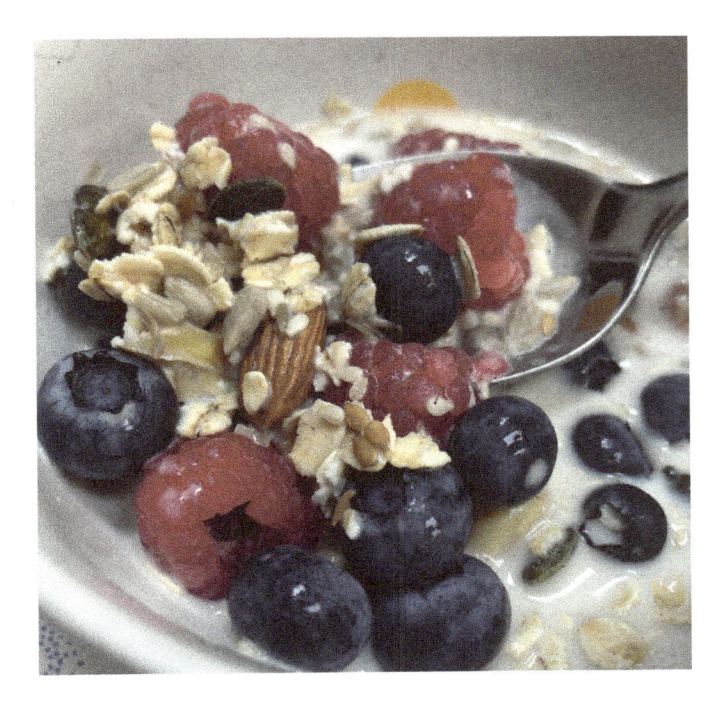

Bircher muesli

Serves 1

Prepare this the night before – make individual portions in glass tumblers.

Measure out enough muesli in a glass tumbler to fill half the glass, pour into a bowl and cover with coconut milk (Koko), grate half an apple into the bowl and mix everything together and then put back into the glass, leave in fridge overnight. In the morning serve with fresh berries.

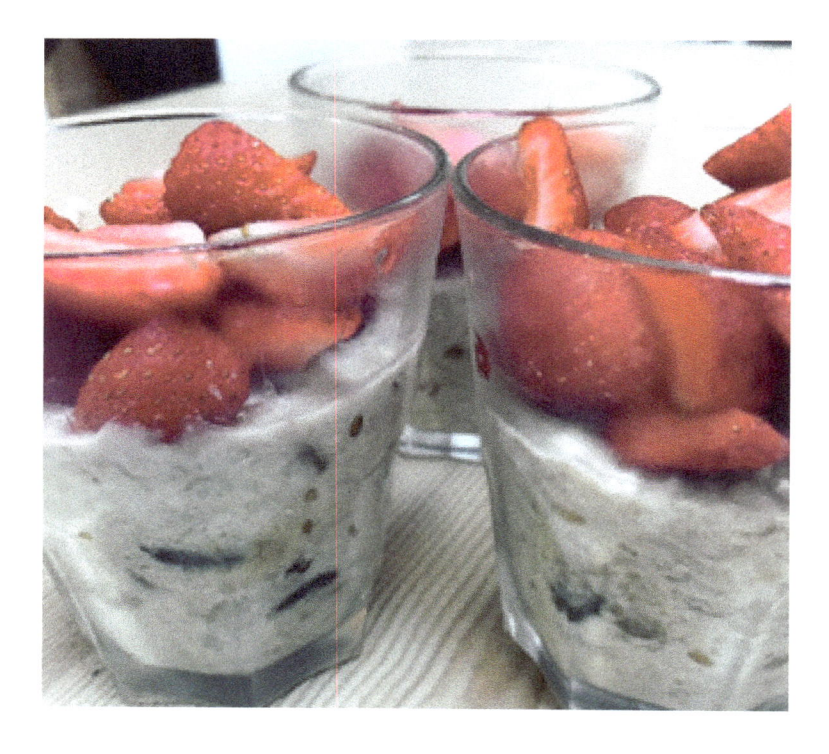

Creamy berry porridge

Serves 2

50g gluten free oats
200ml almond milk (unsweetened)
100ml filtered water
Mixed berries, nuts and seeds, banana slices

Put the oats in a saucepan over a gentle heat, add the milk and water and stir until the porridge is thick and creamy. The longer you cook the oats for, on a gentle heat, the creamier the porridge becomes.

Serve with berries (or add frozen berries with the milk so that they have time to defrost), the sliced banana, nuts and seeds.

You can also try soaking the oats in the milk overnight and then cook the next morning, this process softens the oats and makes them easier to digest.

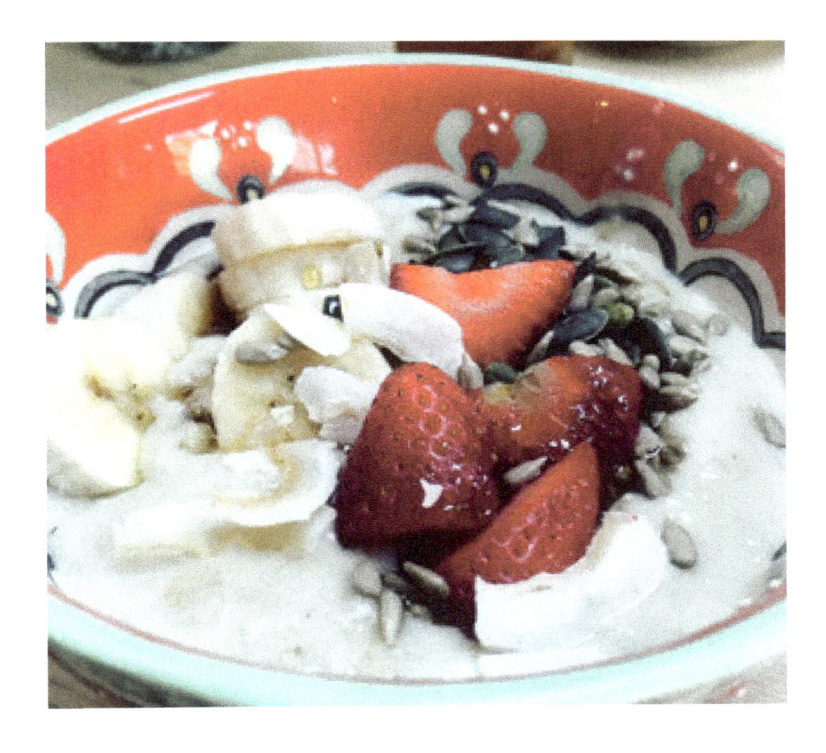

Nutty granola

Serves 1

100g oats
140g walnuts, chopped
140g almonds, chopped
140g hazelnuts, chopped
(or 400g of mixed nuts, chopped - Holland & Barrett sell 400g bags of broken mixed nuts)

140g ground flax seed (Linwoods do good flavours)
100g coconut oil
100g honey or maple syrup
1/2 tbsp cinnamon
1 tbsp vanilla extract (Nielson-Massey)
handful mixed dried fruit, chopped (optional)

Preheat oven to 180°C.

In a big bowl, combine oats, nuts and flaxseed.

In a saucepan, blend together, oil, honey, and cinnamon and heat gently until the mixture starts to bubble. Remove from the heat, add vanilla and stir. Pour over oat mixture and mix well.

Thinly spread on baking sheet(s). Bake until golden approx 15 minutes. Keep an eye on the granola as it cooks as it can easily burn. Cool thoroughly. Add the dried fruit if using. Store in an air tight container.

To make the Almond and Seedy Granola – replace mixed nuts with 250g almonds and 150g mixed seeds.

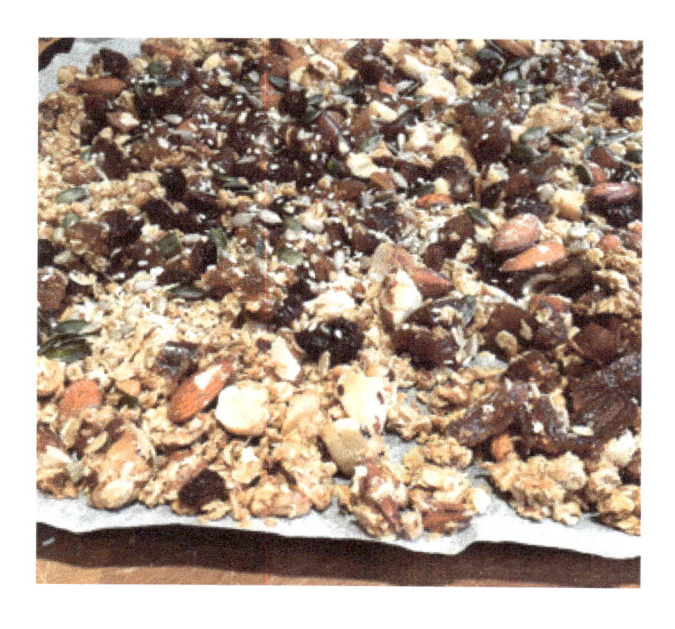

Bread and crackers

These are so delicious there is a definite danger that you will overeat them – don't go crazy and try and restrict yourself to one or two slices of the bread or just a few of the crackers!

Nutty seed bread

This is a very filling gluten free bread full of nuts and seeds – it takes longer to break down in the gut than regular bread made with flour and consequently you feel fuller for longer. The husks and chia seeds provide plenty of soluble fibre which helps to speed transit time. Too much can have a laxative effect!

Please note the dough needs to rest for a minimum of three hours before baking, if you try and cook it without waiting the bread will not hold together. I like to leave the bread in the tin overnight and bake first thing in the morning.

140g sunflower seeds
100g ground flax seeds
70g hazelnuts/almonds
150g gluten free rolled oats
2 tbsp chia seeds

4 tbsp psyllium seed husks
1 tsp sea salt
1 tbsp maple syrup
3 tbsp olive oil or melted coconut oil
350ml water

Combine all the dry ingredients in a bowl. Whisk together the liquid ingredients in a jug: maple syrup, oil and water. Pour this mixture into the dry ingredients and mix thoroughly to form a stiff dough. Spoon the dough into a lined 2lb loaf tin and smooth out.

Leave in the tin for a minimum of three hours or overnight so that the psyllium husks completely absorb all the water.

Preheat oven to 175°C. Place loaf tin in the oven on the middle rack, and bake for 20 minutes. Remove bread from loaf tin, place it upside down directly on the rack and continue to bake for another 30-40 minutes. The bread is ready when it sounds hollow when tapped. Cool completely on a wire rack before slicing.

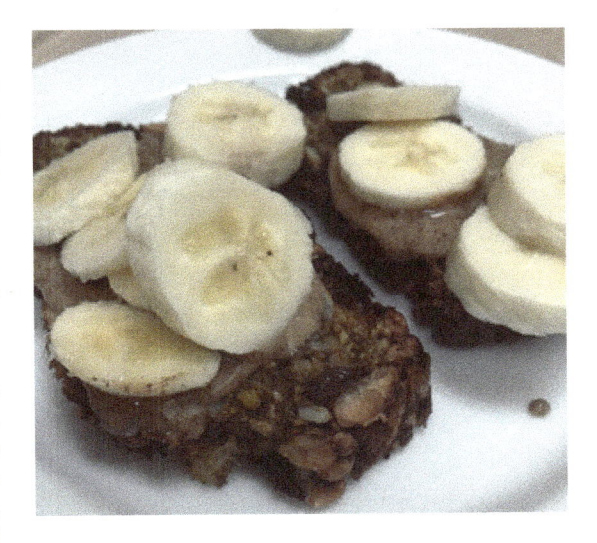

Bread maker fool-proof gluten free bread

My good friend Antonia introduced me to the Panasonic 2500 bread maker a couple of years ago and it has changed my life! I now make a loaf for myself once a week and know I am eating delicious GF bread with no added nasties. I keep the bread wrapped in a tea towel and although it gets drier as the week goes on it is still fine for toasting right to the end.

330ml filtered water
4 tbsp olive oil
1 tbsp maple syrup
1 tsp apple cider vinegar
2 eggs, beaten

450g Doves Farm gluten free bread flour (sold in all big supermarkets in GF section)
1 tsp salt
1 tsp fast acting yeast
100g mixed seeds

Put all the liquid ingredients into the bread maker can and then the dry ingredients on top (adding the yeast last).

Set machine to the GF (Gluten Free) setting with a 'dark crust' – takes 1 hour and 55 mins.

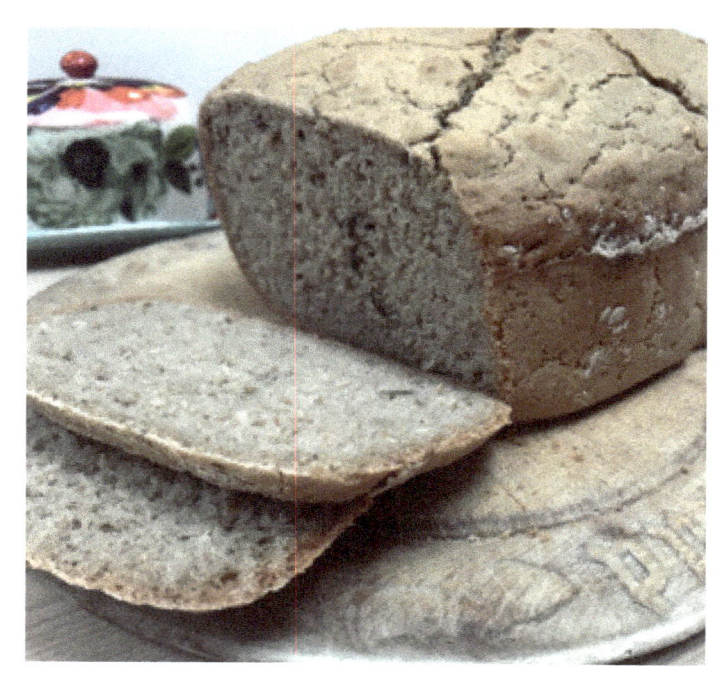

Take out as soon as finished and allow to cool on a wire rack for 20-30 minutes before cutting.

Flax seed crackers

These are a better option than bread if you are trying to reduce the carbohydrate in your diet, they provide plenty of protein and good fats.

100g ground flaxseed (Linwoods have a good range)
100g seeds (try a mixture of sesame, sunflower and pumpkin seeds)
100g gluten free flour (vary with each batch, I like to use quinoa and buckwheat)
olive oil or sundried tomatoes in oil
seasalt or tamari soy sauce
fennel seeds, chilli flakes, caraway seeds, cardamon seeds etc
filtered water – approx. 130ml

Make every batch different by using chopped dried sea vegetables with tamari soy sauce or sundried tomatoes with a little sea salt etc. Invent new crackers every time and you will never get bored of them.

Mix all of the ingredients together with enough water (about 150ml) and a little oil to make a stiff dough. Line 2 baking trays with baking parchment and divide the dough into two portions, placing one on each tray.

Place another layer of baking parchment on top of the first portion of dough and roll it out, between the sheets of parchment, to form a thin layer (2mm thick). Repeat with the other half of dough. Remove the top sheet of parchment and score the crackers to make them easier to break to the correct size after cooking.

Bake in a medium hot oven (180°C) for approx. 20 mins until no longer soft. Keep an eye on the crackers as they catch very easily if you turn your back on them. You may want to turn the crackers mid-way through, removing the paper that was on the underside. Cool on a wire rack, when cold break into crackers.

Store in an airtight tin.

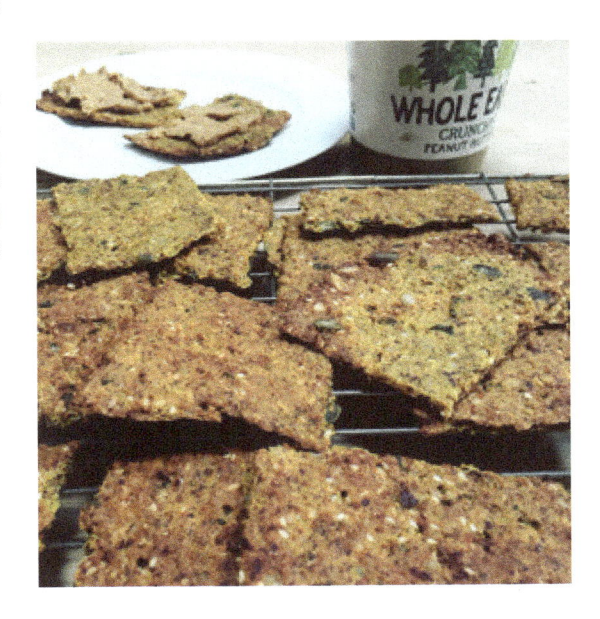

Smashed avocado with chilli and lime

I love this as a breakfast-in-bed treat or actually as a snack anytime, for a more hearty breakfast serve with a poached egg on top.

Serves 1

1 small, ripe avocado
chilli flakes
sea salt and black pepper
half a small lime
2 slices of gluten free bread, toasted

Smash the avocado flesh in a small bowl with a fork. Add a pinch of chilli flakes, a squeeze of lime juice, some sea salt and black pepper. Spread the mixture on the toast.

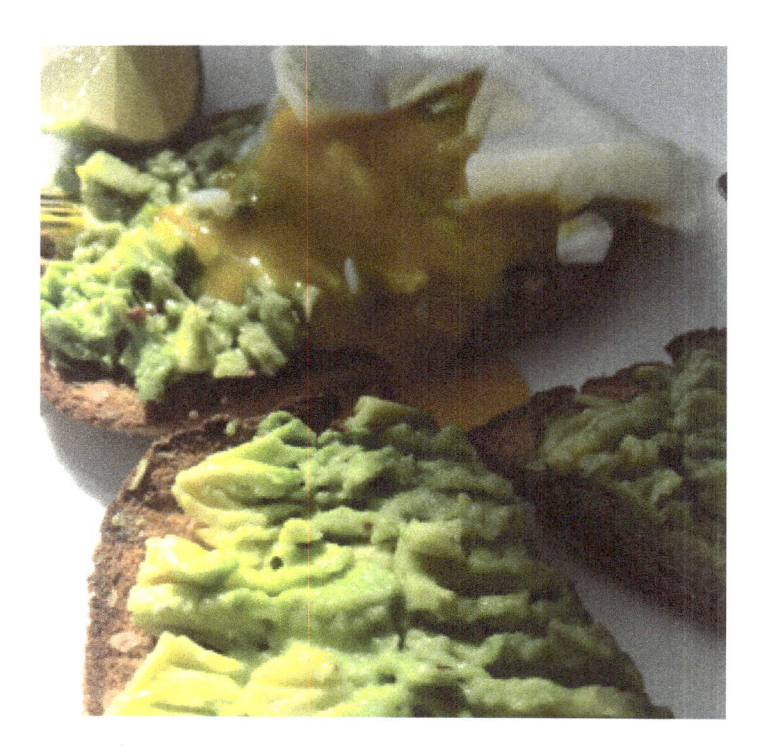

Smoked fish paté

This is going in my breakfast section as clients are always interested in how they can get more protein in at breakfast time, but smoked mackerel and smoked salmon paté are equally delicious at lunch time or on a cracker as an afternoon snack.

200g smoked salmon or smoked mackerel
100g silken tofu or cottage cheese
juice of 1 lemon
freshly ground black pepper
half tsp horseradish

Put all the ingredients into a food processor, season with pepper and blend to a not quite smooth texture. You can make this paté without the tofu/cottage cheese but it will have a drier consistency.

This recipe works well with smoked trout too.

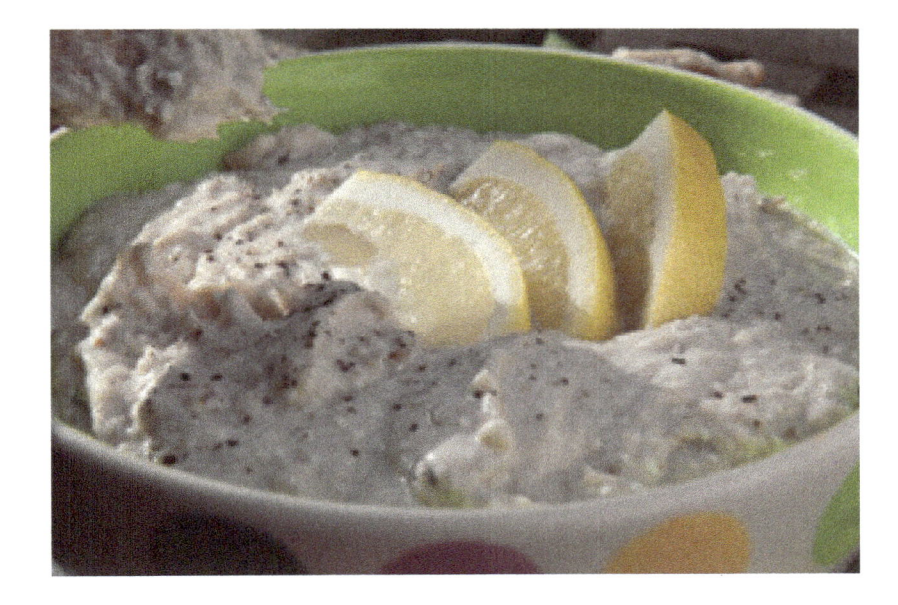

Pancakes

Pancakes are great when you have a little more time, but if you are super organized pancakes are great any day of the week. Serve with: berries and yoghurt, berries and tahini, chopped fruit, avocado, smoked salmon ....

Buckwheat pancakes

Serves 4

200g buckwheat flour
2 eggs
2 tsp cinnamon
zest and juice of 1 orange
2 tsp baking powder (gluten free)
soya/Koko or almond milk (approx 250ml)
coconut oil

Mix flour, cinnamon, zest and baking powder in a large bowl. Add eggs and juice and gradually beat in the milk until the mixture forms a batter with a dropping consistency (coats the back of a spoon but still pourable).

Put a heavy based frying pan on the heat. Melt the coconut oil (1 tsp) to cover the bottom of the pan, pour off any excess. Pour a ladleful of the batter into the pan and cook for 2-3mins until bubbles appear, flip over and cook for another 2 mins. until golden. Repeat until all the batter has been used, using more coconut oil as necessary.

Alternatively the batter keeps well in the fridge in a sealed jar for up to 3 days.

To make these vegan: 1 tbsp of ground flax seed mixed with 3 tbsp of water makes a good egg substitute (so use 2 tbsp seeds with 6 tbsp water for this recipe).

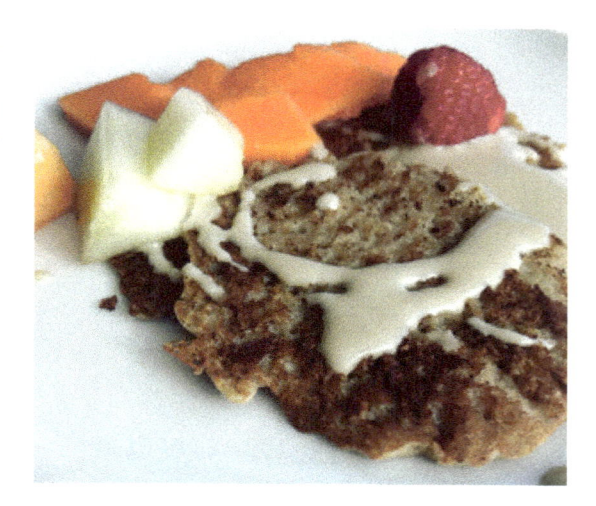

Almond and coconut pancakes

Serves 2 (2 pancakes each)

2 tbsp ground almonds
2 tbsp coconut flour
2 eggs

4 tbsp sparkling water
pinch of salt
coconut oil for cooking

Mix all ingredients together in a bowl until there are no lumps . Heat a teaspoon of coconut oil in a frying pan. Use a 1/4 cup measure to spoon mixture into the pan and look for bubbling or browning of the edges before flipping. Serve with toppings of your choice.

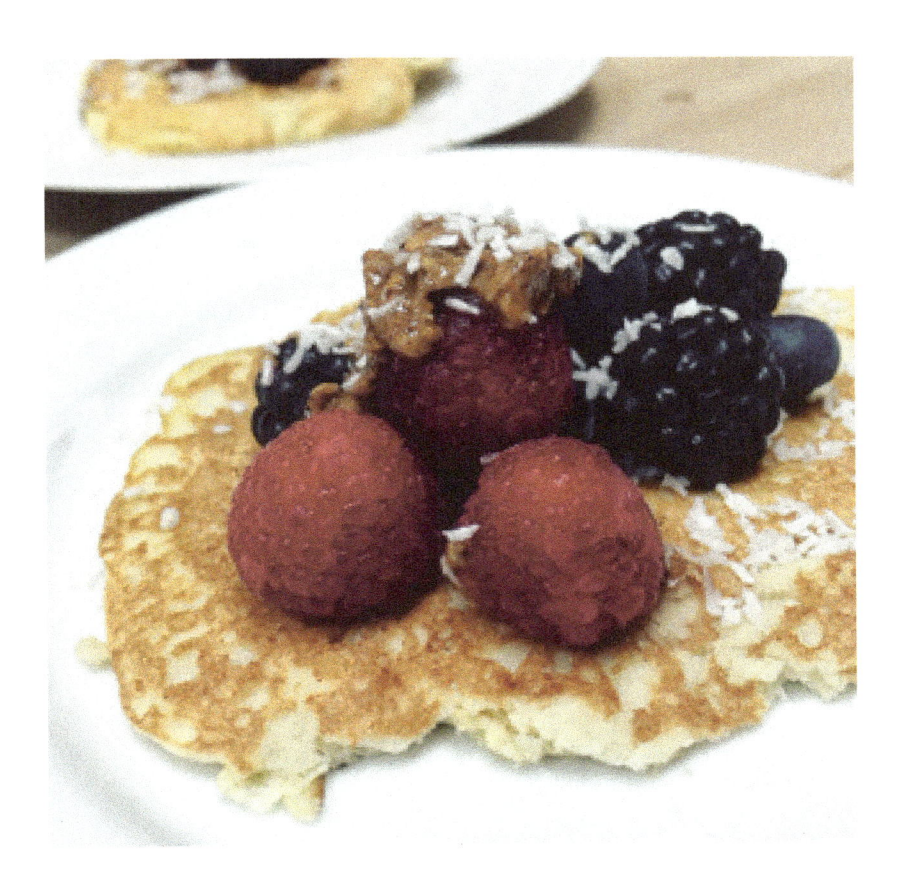

Home-made baked beans

Serves 2

extra virgin olive oil
half an onion, finely chopped
1 clove of garlic, finely chopped
1 tbsp tomato purée
half tsp smoked paprika
half tsp fresh thyme leaves

1 tsp coconut sugar
1 tsp tamari soy sauce
400g can cannellini beans
200g passata
a handful of spinach leaves (optional)
sea salt & freshly ground black pepper

Sauté the onion and garlic in a tablespoon of olive oil until softened. Add the tomato purée, paprika, thyme, sugar and tamari soy sauce and simmer for a few minutes.

Add the drained beans and passata and continue to simmer until the liquid around the beans has reduced and thickened. Season with salt and black pepper.

Add the spinach and stir so that it wilts into the beans.

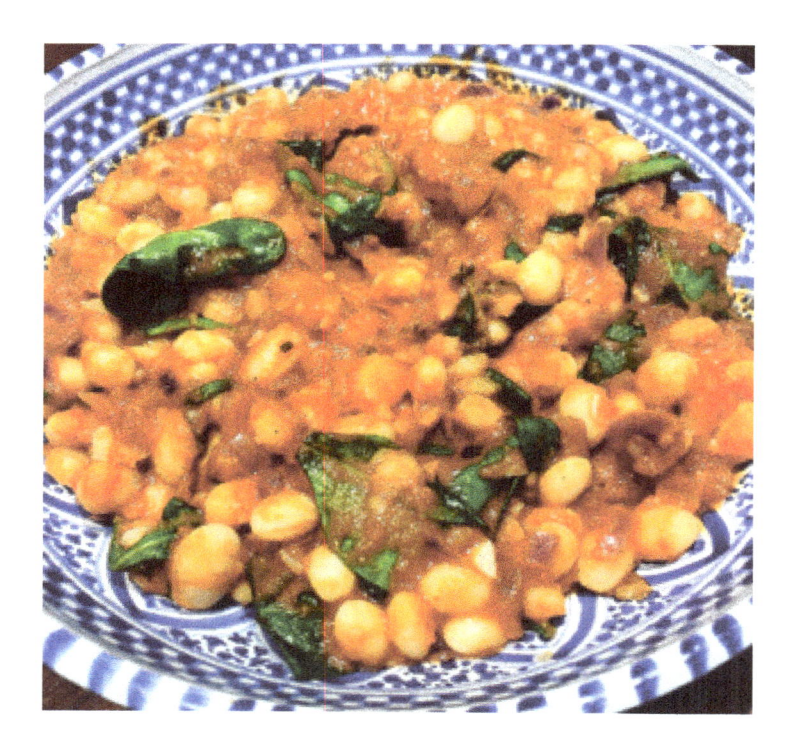

Soups

Soups tend to be easy to digest, simple to make and a good way to get more vegetables into your diet. Never throw away a chicken carcass as you can easily turn it into a tasty stock for soups. As a vegetarian option I use Marigold bouillon for making stock.

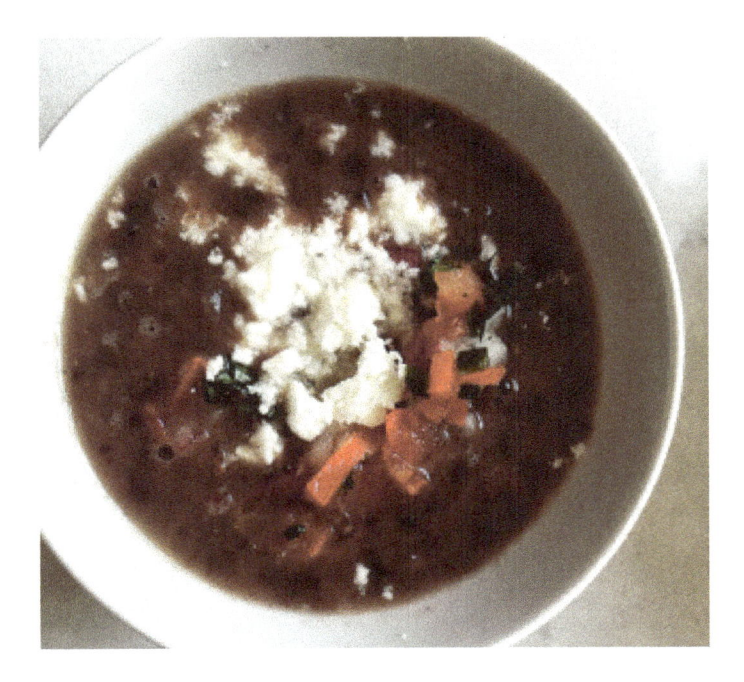

Easy chicken stock

1 chicken carcass
2 bay leaves
1 onion
1 carrot

1 celery heart
mixed herbs
sea salt & black pepper

Put all the ingredients in a large saucepan and cover with water. Bring to the boil and simmer for approx. 3 hours until you have a tasty stock.

Sieve to remove the bones and vegetables and keep in the fridge or freezer ready for your next soup.

Mum's chicken soup

2 tbsp olive oil
2 medium onions, chopped
2 cloved garlic, chopped
3 carrots, chopped
1 tbsp thyme leaves

1.5 litres chicken stock
200g red lentils, rinsed
300g leftover roast chicken, shredded
200g green vegetables of your choice: broccoli, green beans, frozen peas etc.

Heat the olive oil in a large, heavy based saucepan. Add the onion, carrots, garlic and thyme and gently cook for about 10 mins.

Stir in the chicken stock and lentils, bring to the boil and simmer for 15 mins until the lentils are soft. Add the chicken and green vegetables and continue to simmer until the vegetables are tender.

Season well and serve.

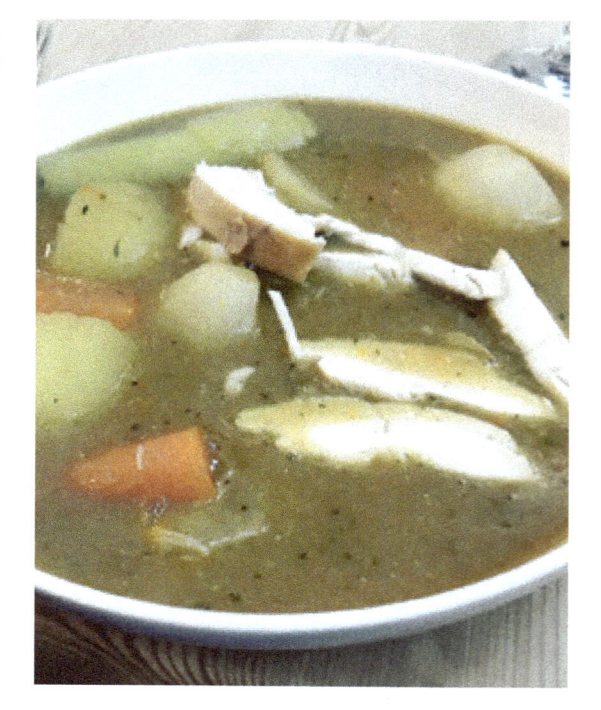

Lentil, spinach and tomato soup

This was in my first book and has become a staple for lots of my friends and clients.

Serves 6

2 carrots, peeled and sliced
2 sticks celery, sliced
2 medium onions, peeled & chopped
2 cloves garlic, peeled & sliced
extra virgin olive oil
3cm piece of fresh ginger
1 fresh red chilli

10 cherry tomatoes
1.8 litres of stock, Marigold Bouillon
or fresh chicken stock
300g red lentils
200g spinach
sea salt & freshly ground black pepper

Heat a large pan and add 2 tablespoons of olive oil. Add the carrots, celery, onions and garlic and cook for approx 10 mins with the lid askew, until the carrots are softened. Meanwhile peel and grate the ginger, deseed and slice the chilli finely and slice the tomatoes in half.

Add the stock to the pan with the lentils, ginger, chilli and tomatoes. Bring the soup to the boil and then reduce the heat and simmer for approx 10 mins with the lid on until the lentils are cooked. Add the spinach and let it wilt into the soup. Season as necessary and serve immediately.

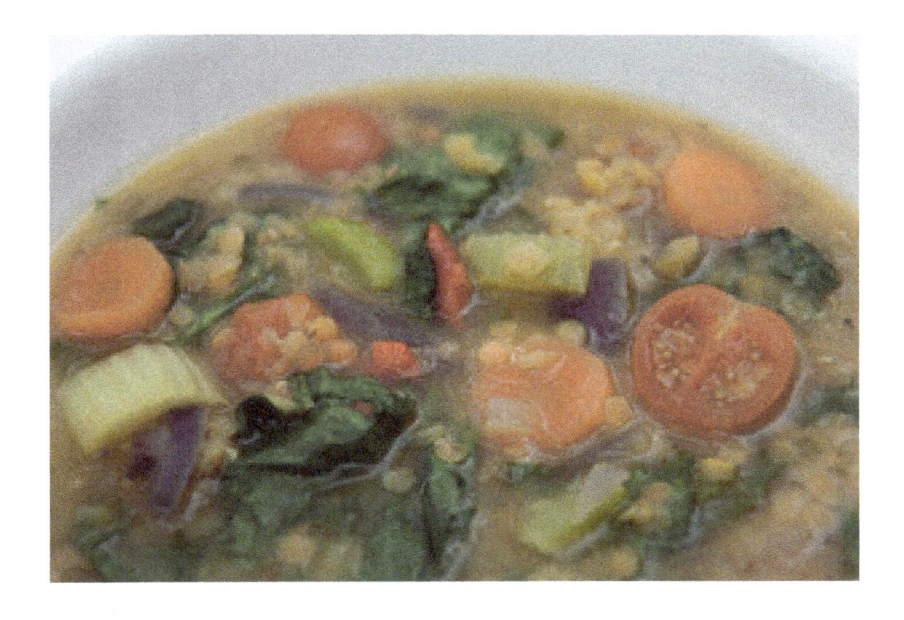

Roasted butternut squash soup

If you have time roast the butternut squash before making this soup as it gives the soup a more velvety texture.

Serves 4

3 tbsp olive oil
1 red onion chopped
1 large garlic clove, chopped
600ml water
750g butternut squash, peeled weight – deseeded and chopped (if time roasted: arrange chunks in a single layer on a baking tray, drizzle with olive oil and season then roast in the oven for 30mins)

1 large carrot, chopped
2 tsp Marigold bouillion
1 red chilli, deseeded & chopped
1 tsp finely grated fresh ginger
1 tsp lemon juice

Heat the oil in a large pan, add the onion and garlic and cook gently for 5 mins until soft. Add the squash and carrot and cook gently for another 5 mins. Add water and bouillon, bring to boil and simmer for 15 mins. Add the red chilli, ginger and lemon juice and simmer for another 15 mins.

Blend until smooth with a hand blender and serve.

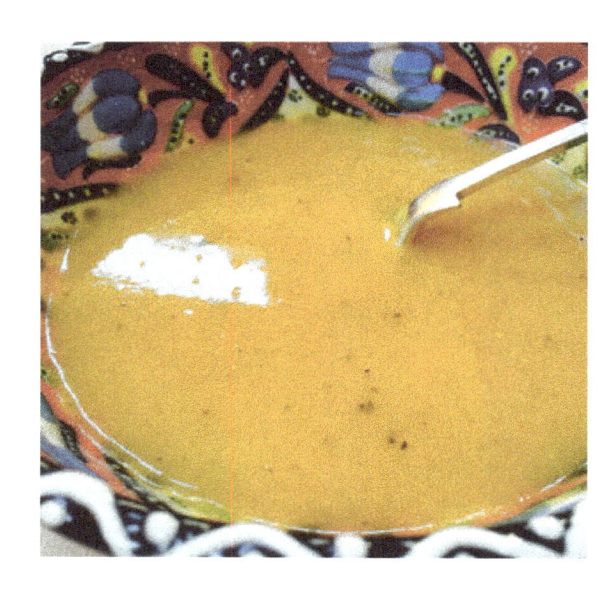

Roasted red pepper soup

When I have more time I roast 5 red peppers in the oven for 30 mins instead of using peppers from a jar. Once out of the oven put the peppers in a Pyrex bowl and cover with clingfilm so that they steam, allow to cool for a little and then remove skins and core/seeds. This takes time but the soup tastes even better.

Serves 4

280g jar of red peppers, drained and finely sliced
2 tbsp olive oil
1 onion, finely diced
2 cloves garlic, crushed
1 tsp cumin seeds, ground
1 tsp fresh thyme leaves
1 tsp smoked Spanish paprika
200g red lentils, rinsed
400g can chopped tomatoes
1.2 litres vegetables stock
2 tbsp of finely chopped parsley
salt to taste
juice of 1-2 lemons

Sauté the onion in the oil until soft, add the garlic, cumin and thyme, then add the paprika, lentils, tomatoes and stock. Simmer. Add the peppers to the soup and continue to cook until the lentils start to break down.

Stir in the parsley and season with salt and lemon juice adding some extra paprika if necessary and a swirl of extra virgin olive oil as you serve.

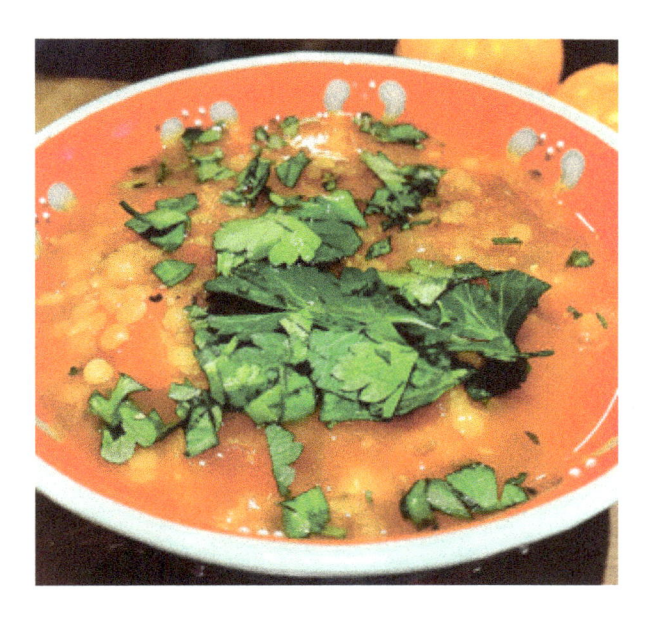

Pear and fennel soup

I was a bit dubious when I first experimented with this soup but you should try it, so delicious and just a handful of ingredients.

Serves 4

2 large fennel bulbs, trimmed
2 tbsp olive oil
2 onions
2 garlic cloves, finely chopped

1.2 litres vegetables stock made with Marigold bouillon
2 pears, peeled, cored and chopped

Chop the fennel bulbs. Heat the olive oil in a large saucepan and sauté the onion and garlic. Add the fennel and pears and the stock, bring to the boil and then reduce heat to a simmer for 40 mins.

Blend with a hand blender until smooth.

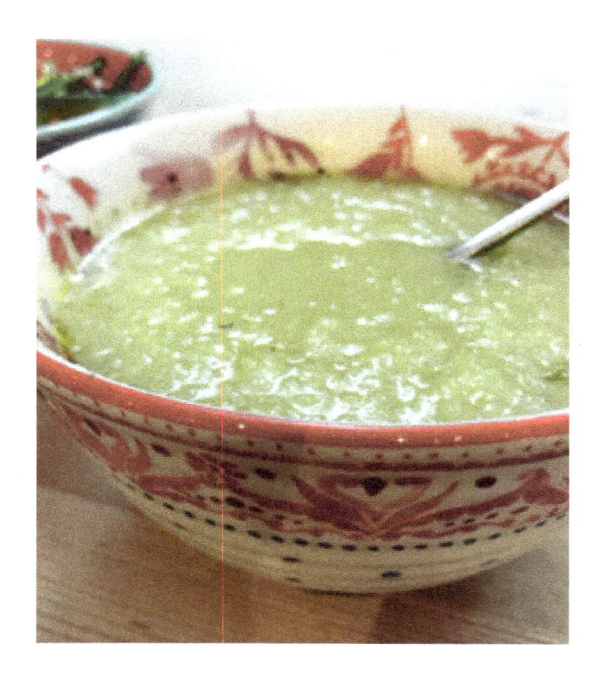

Mexican black bean soup with fresh tomato salsa

I originally made this soup for a Mexican themed Cookery Workshop and was really flattered when one of the participants, who happened to be Mexican, said that this soup reminded him of his mother's cooking. I have wowed guests with it at dinner parties and it continues to be a family favourite. Thoroughly recommended!

Chipotles en adobe paste comes in a jar and you can find it in large supermarkets or online – if you really can't find it then substitute one finely chopped fresh red chilli or a teaspoon of harissa paste.

Serves 4

2 plum tomatoes
3 garlic cloves, unpeeled
25g butter
olive oil
1 small white onion, finely chopped
1 tbsp fresh oregano, chopped
2 fresh bay leaves

1 tsp Chipotles en adobo (available from Sainsbury's or online from The Cool Chile Company)
sea salt & freshly ground black pepper
2 cans/cartons of black beans, drained
1 litre stock (Marigold bouillon)
juice of 1 lime

Dry roast the tomatoes and garlic in a heavy based frying pan until blackened, then remove the skins.

Meanwhile, heat the butter and a tbsp of oil in a large, heavy based pan and when the butter foams add the onion, oregano and bay leaves. Sweat for about 10 mins. and then add the garlic. Cook for a few minutes before adding the skinned tomatoes and Chipotle paste. Season well with salt and pepper. Cook gently for a few minutes and then add the drained beans, the stock and lime juice. Simmer for about another 10 mins.

Whizz with a hand blender – briefly for a textured soup, longer for a smooth soup. Pour the soup into bowls, add some salsa and perhaps a crumble of feta.

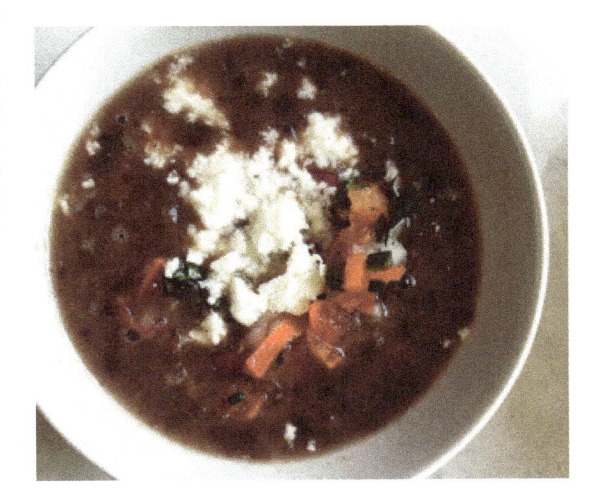

Fresh tomato salsa

4 large tomatoes, finely chopped (seeds removed)
1 small red onion, finely chopped
1 green chilli, finely chopped

juice of 1 lime
small handful coriander leaves, chopped
1 tbsp olive oil
sea salt & black pepper

Combine all of the ingredients to make delicious salsa that actually goes with everything!

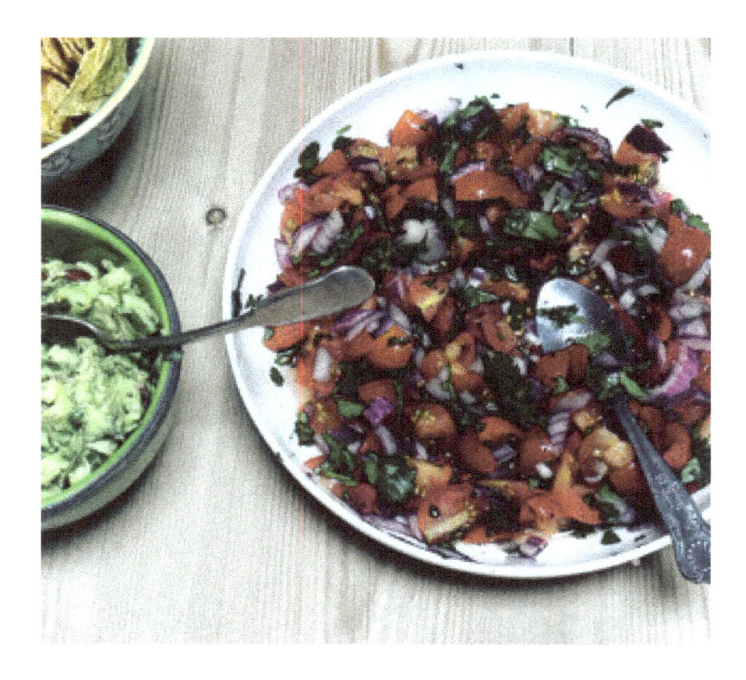

Bissara broad bean soup

This is another soup that I experimented with for a cookery workshop, a Moroccan themed event. The key is to cook this quickly and serve immediately – a soup in under 10 minutes!

Serves 4

500g frozen baby broad beans
1 litre boiling water
6 garlic cloves
3 tsp Marigold bouillion stock powder
1 tsp sea salt

3 tbsp extra virgin olive oil
1 tsp ground cumin
1 tsp paprika
chopped fresh mint

Dissolve the Marigold stock powder in the boiling water in a jug, add to a saucepan with the broad beans, garlic cloves and sea salt and simmer for approx 4-5 mins.

Meanwhile in a small bowl stir the paprika and cumin into the olive oil.

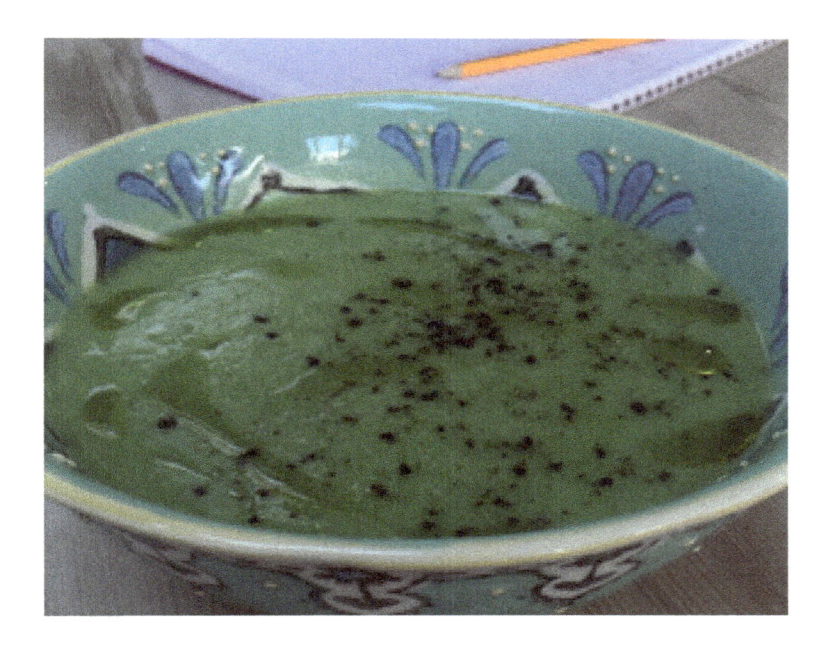

Blitz the soup with a hand blender until smooth. Drizzle with the oil mix and add mint to serve.

Tom Yum soup with noodles

This is an all time favourite from my original book but it's a recipe I go back to time and time again.

Serves 4

1 litre of light stock, made with Marigold bouillion
6 small sticks lemongrass
12 ripped lime leaves
1 long red chilli, sliced
20g fresh ginger, thinly sliced
2 tbsp fish sauce

20g palm sugar (or dark brown sugar)
200g precooked tiger prawns (optional)
handful coriander leaves
handful Thai basil leaves
2 limes, halved
200g buckwheat or rice noodles

Heat the stock in a large pan and add the lemongrass, torn lime leaves, chilli, ginger, fish sauce and sugar. Bring to the boil, then reduce the heat to very low and leave to infuse for 10 minutes. Meanwhile you can cook your noodles in a saucepan of boiling water – drain them and run cold water over them to stop them from overcooking. Drop the prawns into the broth, and heat through for a couple of minutes.

Put a little coriander and basil into the bottom of four bowls, along with a serving of noodles. Squeeze a little lime juice over the top and pour in the hot soup. Serve with a wedge of lime.

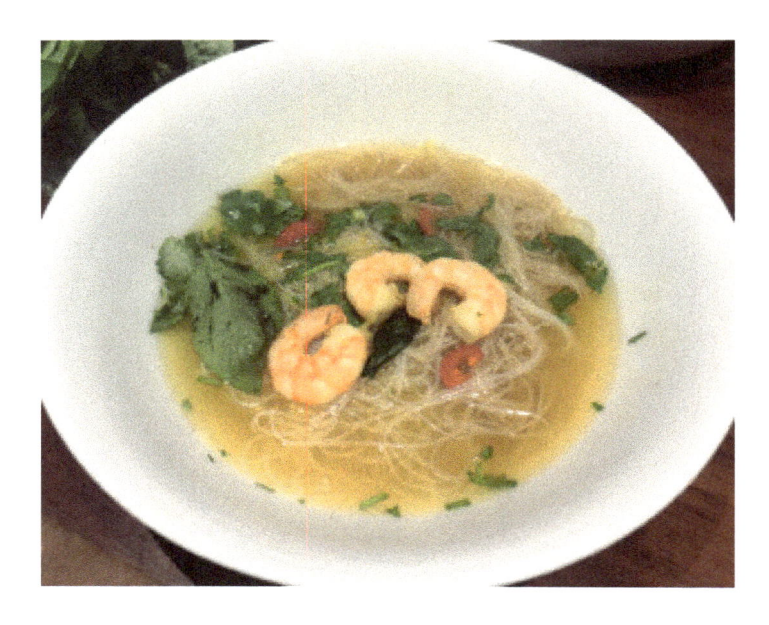

Thai laksa with tofu and prawns

I deliberated over whether this should go in the soup or the mains section as we often have it as the main event for dinner but I decided that as it is most definitely a soup it should go here.

I can't stop making this, sometimes with tofu, sometimes prawns and sometimes with both. My family love it, it tastes so authentically Thai yet is easy and quick to make – perfect.

Serves 4

300g Thai flat rice noodles
300g tofu, cut into cubes
2 tbsp olive oil
4 garlic cloves, peeled
5cm piece of ginger, peeled
2 red chillies, deseeded
2 tbsp fish sauce
2 tbsp tamari soy sauce
1 tsp ground turmeric

2 tsp coconut palm sugar
or dark brown sugar
2 limes, juiced
2 400g cans of coconut milk
1 250g bag of large cooked
king prawns, defrosted
coriander, to serve
100g beansprouts, to serve

Rinse the rice noodles in cold water and place them in a large bowl, covered with plenty of boiling water. Leave to soften – 5-10 minutes depending on the brand. Drain and rinse under running cold water to stop them from going too soft.

Heat the olive oil in a wok and then stir fry the cubed tofu until golden.

Blitz the garlic, ginger and chillies in a food processor along with the fish sauce, soy sauce, turmeric, sugar and lime juice. Heat this mixture for a couple of minutes in a large heavy based pan until fragrant. Add the coconut milk plus 200ml of water and simmer for 5 mins. Add the tofu and prawns to heat through.

Divide the noodles between bowls and ladle over the hot laksa. Top with coriander and beansprouts and serve.

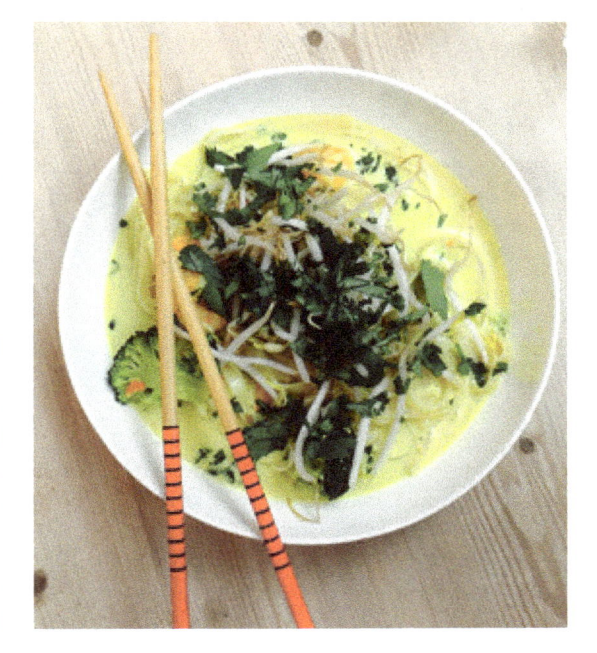

Butternut miso soup with soba noodles

This is adapted from a recipe from one of my favourite books 'My New Roots', to increase the protein in this meal I sometimes add a fillet of pan fried salmon per serving which makes it incredibly satisfying.

Serves 4

1 tbsp coconut oil
2 medium white onions
¾ tsp sea salt
3 cloves garlic
1kg butternut squash
750ml – 1 litre water
3 – 4 tbsp sweet white miso paste
1 tbsp grated fresh ginger
175g soba noodles (100% buckwheat) or black rice noodles

toppings:
spring onion
sesame seeds
sautéed mushrooms (shitake work well)
Nori seaweed in fine strips

Roughly chop the onions and garlic. Wash the squash and chop into chunks – no need to peel.

In a large saucepan, melt the coconut oil or use olive oil. Add the onions and salt, stir to coat and cook for about 10 minutes until the onions are just starting to caramelize. Add the garlic and cook for another minute. Add the squash and stir to coat. Add 750ml of water, cover, bring to a boil, and reduce to a simmer for about 15 mins, until the squash is tender.

While the soup is cooking, prepare the toppings: Bring a pot of salted water to the boil. Cook the soba noodles according to packet directions, drain and lightly rinse in cold water. Slice spring onion, lightly toast sesame seeds in a dry skillet over a medium heat, about 2-3 minutes. Sauté mushrooms in a lightly oiled pan for 5-7 mins.

Use a hand blender to blitz the soup until completely smooth. Add more water if necessary – for a creamy but not too thin consistency. Add the miso paste and ginger and blend again until smooth. Season as necessary.

Ladle the soup into bowls, top with soba, spring onion, sesame seeds, mushrooms and arrange the seaweed over top. Serve immediately.

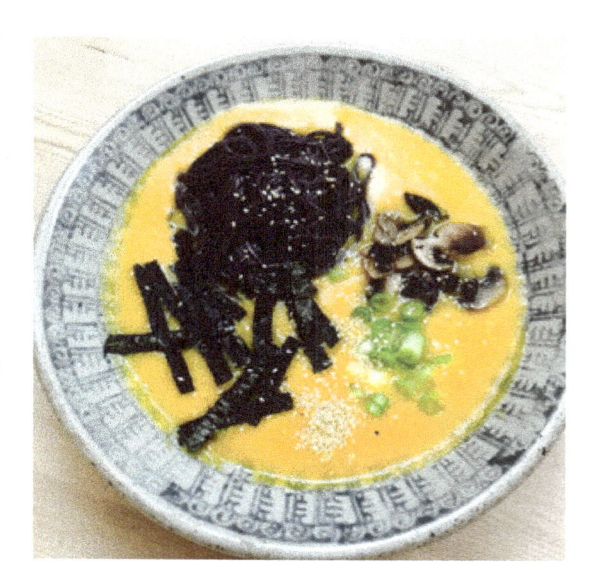

Minestrone soup

It is worth making a vat of this and freezing it in portions as there is quite a lot of chopping involved but it is so worth it! You could make this a lighter soup in Summer by using French beans, broad beans and peas (added at same time as tomatoes) instead of the squash and carrot.

Serves 4

2 tbsp olive oil
1 onion
1 leek
2 celery sticks
2 carrots
200g butternut squash or pumpkin
1 garlic clove, finely chopped
sprig thyme

1 tbsp chopped sage
1 can/jar of borlotti or cannellini beans
1 litre Marigold boullion stock
400g can of tomatoes
200g cavolo nero leaves or spinach
sea salt & ground black pepper
Engevita nutritional yeast flakes/
grated fresh Parmesan cheese

Dice the onion, leek, celery, squash and carrot to same size pieces. Slice cavolo nero leaves/spinach into strips.

Heat the olive oil in large pan and add the onions, leeks, celery, squash, carrot and garlic, sauté until soft. Add the thyme, sage and beans and sauté for further 2mins.
Add the stock and can of tomatoes and bring to the boil, simmer until vegetables are tender.

Lastly add the spinach/cavolo nero leaves, season and serve with Engevita nutritional yeast flakes for a non-dairy (vegan) cheesy taste or with grated Parmesan cheese.

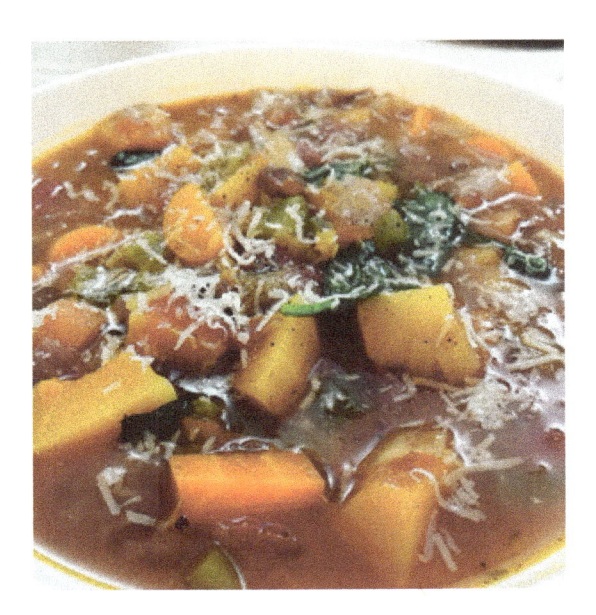

Veggie sides

I am always telling people that half of their plate should be made up of vegetables as so many people add them as an afterthought whereas veggies should really be the main focus. Learning how to make some of these side dishes will really help with this – no effort at all – I could eat the Moroccan Dip all day!

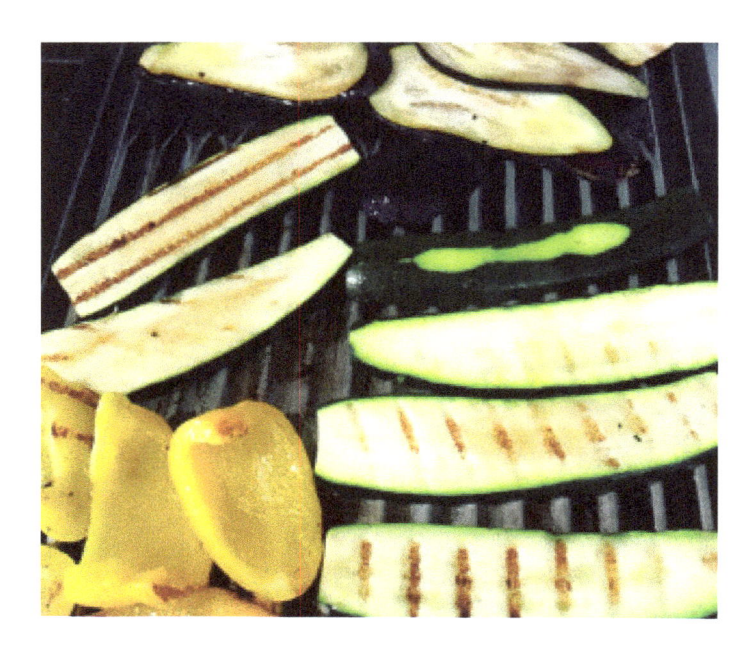

Moroccan beetroot dip

I often make this when friends are coming over – always hoping there will be some over to add to my salad the following day!

Serves 4

2 x 250g packets of cooked beetroot in natural juice (or 4 home-cooked large beetroots)
1 garlic clove, crushed to a paste with a little salt
4 tbsp extra virgin olive oil

4 tbsp thick yoghurt
2 tbsp chopped dill
2 tbsp red wine vinegar
50g feta cheese, crumbled
walnut halves, broken
half tsp black onion seeds

Blend the beetroot in a food processor, leaving some texture – not too smooth. In a shallow bowl combine the beetroot with the garlic, olive oil, yoghurt, dill, vinegar and a pinch more salt, mix. Sprinkle with the feta, walnuts and onion seeds and drizzle with a little more olive oil.

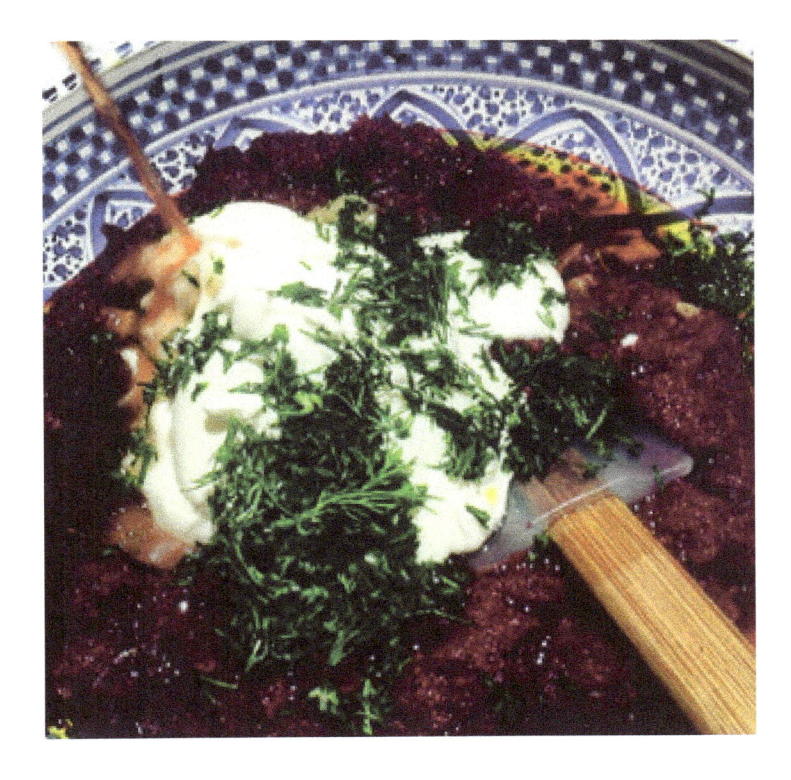

Aubergine three ways:
Aubergine with miso dressing

Serves 4

2 medium aubergines
1 tsp coconut oil, melted or olive oil

dressing:
2 tbsp sweet white miso (Clearspring)
1 tbsp brown rice vinegar
1 tsp pure maple syrup
1 tbsp tahini
2 tbsp sesame seeds
3 tbsp chives, chopped

Preheat oven to 200°C. Line a baking sheet with baking parchment.

Slice the aubergines in half lengthwise. Score the flesh on the diagonal and rub in a little coconut/olive oil. Put the aubergine halves, cut side up, on the baking sheet and bake until golden – about 20 mins.

Meanwhile whisk the miso, vinegar, maple syrup and tahini together in a small bowl. Toast the sesame seeds in a dry pan for 5 mins until fragrant.

Remove the aubergines from the oven and spread evenly with the miso glaze, using a spatula. Sprinkle with the toasted sesame seeds. Grill the aubergines for a couple of minutes until brown. Sprinkle with chives and serve.

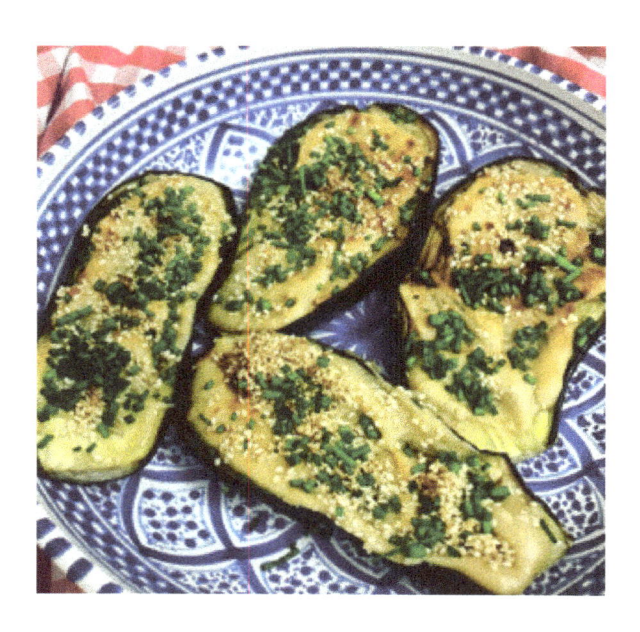

Aubergine with tahini dressing

Serves 2

1 large aubergine
olive oil or melted coconut oil
coarse sea salt
pomegranate seeds
1 tbsp date syrup or pomegranate molasses
mint leaves, roughly chopped

dressing:
2 tbsp tahini
6-8 tbsp boiling water
half a small garlic, finely chopped
150g natural yoghurt
3 tbsp freshly squeezed lemon juice
3 tbsp olive oil
half tsp sea salt
quarter tsp black pepper

(this makes twice as much as you will need – but good to have in fridge)

Preheat oven to 200°C and line a baking tray with parchment paper.

Slice the aubergine in half lengthwise. Score the flesh on the diagonal, sprinkle with sea salt and rub in a little coconut/olive oil. Put the aubergine halves, cut side up, on the baking sheet and bake until golden – about 20 mins.

Meanwhile whisk the tahini and water together to form a smooth paste. Whisk in rest of ingredients.

Transfer the aubergine to a platter. Drizzle it with the dressing and then with date syrup. Scatter the mint and pomegranate seeds over the top – serve warm or cold.

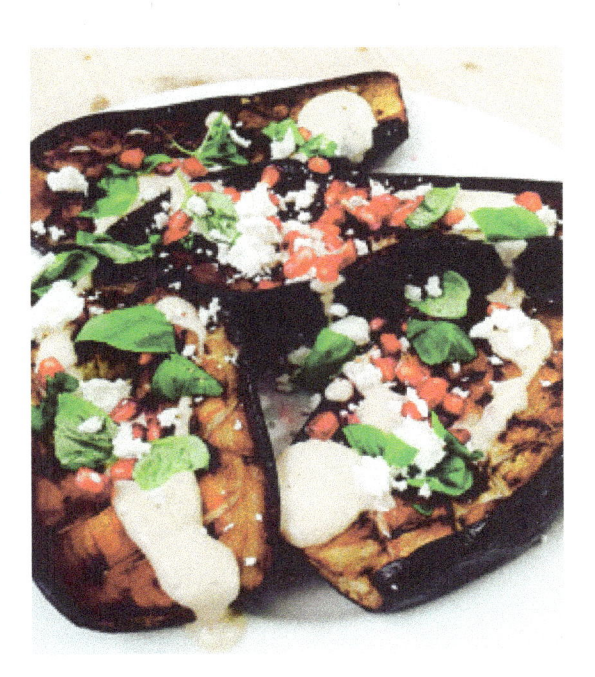

Sticky and spicy aubergine

Great with grilled lamb and humous but it would work well with roast chicken or pan fried white fish.

Serves 4

2 large aubergines, cut into 1cm thick rounds and drizzled with olive oil
1 heaped tbsp rose harissa
1 tbsp maple syrup
1 tsp sesame seeds
1 tsp nigella seeds
small bunch coriander, chopped
2 spring onions, thinly sliced in rounds

Heat a griddle and grill the oiled aubergines on both sides until cooked through and golden. In a shallow bowl combine the harissa with maple syrup and add the aubergine rounds - mixing to ensure they are covered in the mixture. Season with sea salt and some black pepper. Serve with the seeds, coriander and spring onions scattered over the top.

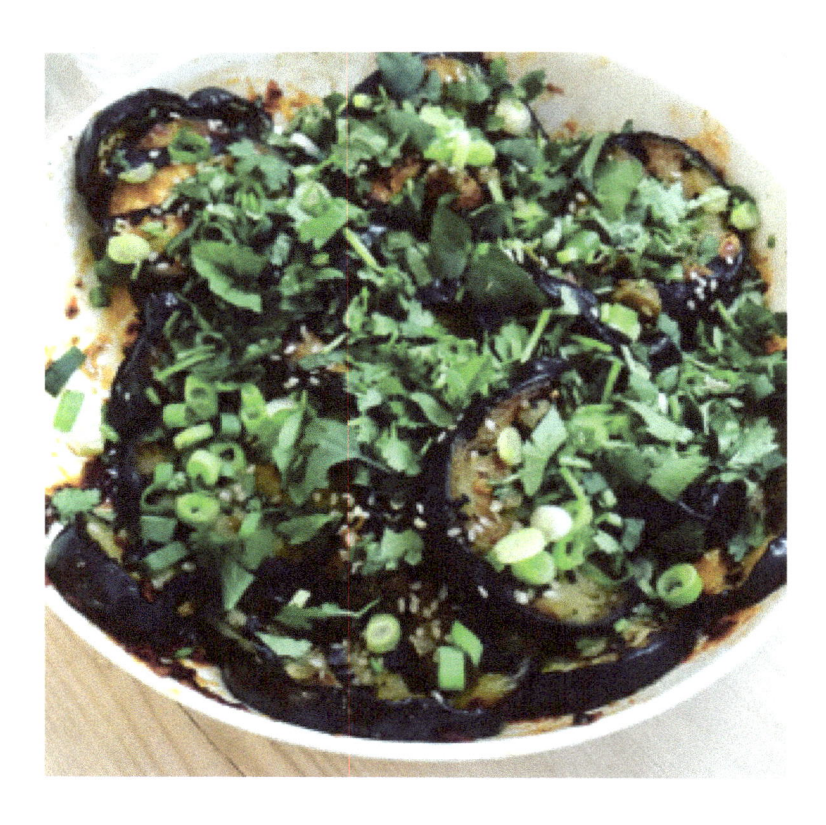

Sauerkraut

Fermented foods can be beneficial for the digestive system - they are thought to be able to increase the level of beneficial bacteria in the gut. My advice is to make your own sauerkraut or kimchi pickles as it is very therapeutic and makes you feel smug and then try a small portion and see how you get on – it doesn't suit everyone but I'm a fan.

300g Savoy cabbage, finely shredded
3 raw beetroots, peeled and very thinly sliced
2 tsp caraway seeds
2 tsp sea salt

In a large bowl rub the salt into the sliced vegetables for at least 10 minutes until they are very limp and wet. Mix in the caraway seeds. Pack the vegetables into a sterilized jar and press down so that the water covers the vegetables, if necessary adding a little filtered water to cover. I use fermenting jars that I bought on Amazon which have a special lid with a sterilock but if you don't have these you can use a smaller weighted jar (filled with marbles or something heavy) to press down on the vegetables to ensure that they stay under the water. Cover with a cloth and secure with a rubber band. Place the jar in a dark cupboard for 3 days, occasionally checking to make sure that water still covers the vegetables and 'tamping' down with the smaller jar to keep the vegetables tightly packed. Once the vegetables have fermented you can then store in the fridge – lasts for weeks.

Experiment with different vegetables, fennel and kohlrabi also work well, actually all vegetables work as long as you slice them very thinly – I use a mandolin to do this – taking the very greatest of care as this is super sharp.

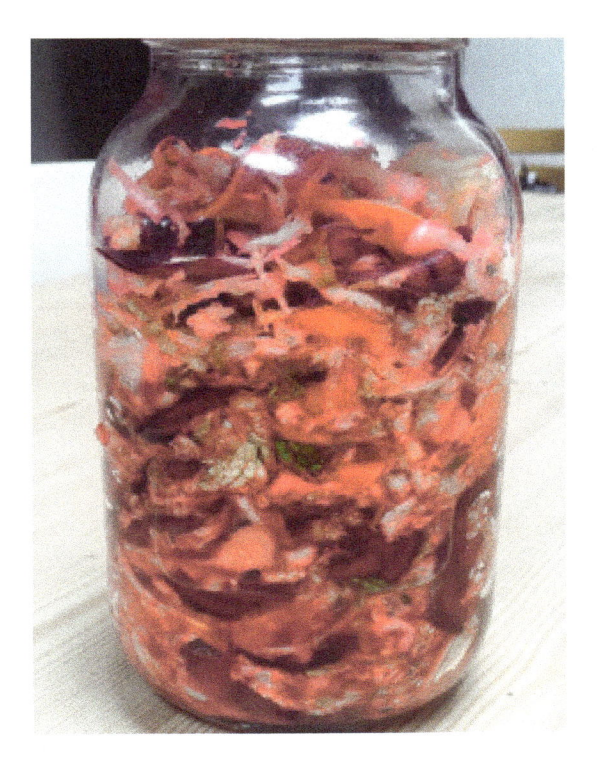

Kimchi pickles

1 savoy cabbage - chopped finely
2 carrots - cut into matchsticks
1 daikon (if you can find one!) chopped into matchsticks or thin rounds
5 spring onions - just the green part finely chopped

1 onion, roughly chopped
1 inch piece of ginger
1 inch piece of fresh turmeric
8 garlic gloves, peeled
red chilli flakes - to taste
sea salt

Weigh the chopped cabbage, carrots, daikon and spring onions, in order to calculate how much salt to use and then place these vegetables in a large bowl.

Blitz the onion, ginger, turmeric, garlic and chilli flakes to a paste in a food processor. Add sea salt – 3 tablespoons per 2kgs of vegetables.

Pour the paste over the chopped vegetables and massage into the vegetables (best to wear latex gloves for this otherwise your hands will be yellow for days!) for at least 10 minutes to release the water from the vegetables. Pack the vegetables into Kilner Jars and either use lids with Steri-Locks (from Amazon) or cover with a cloth and secure with a rubber band.

Keep the jars in a dark cupboard for 4 days before transferring to the fridge. Whilst fermenting check on the pickles every day to make sure that the vegetables are slightly under water level - if not top up with a little mineral water - use a wooden spoon to 'tamp' down the vegetables - keeping it tightly packed down in the jar. After 4 days transfer to the fridge – keeps for ages.

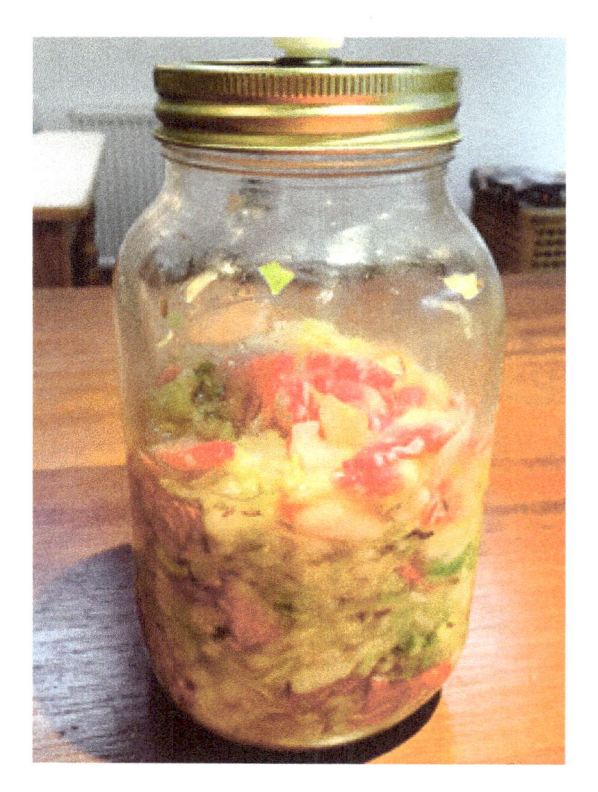

Tempeh

250g tempeh, cut into strips

vinaigrette :
2 tbsp apple cider vinegar
half shallot, chopped
3 tbsp extra virgin olive oil
pinch sea salt

Whisk all the vinaigrette ingredients together in a bowl and add the tempeh. Allow tempeh to marinate in the dressing for 30 minutes (in the fridge) and then arrange it in a single layer on a baking tray and bake in the oven for 15-20 mins until golden, turning half way through.

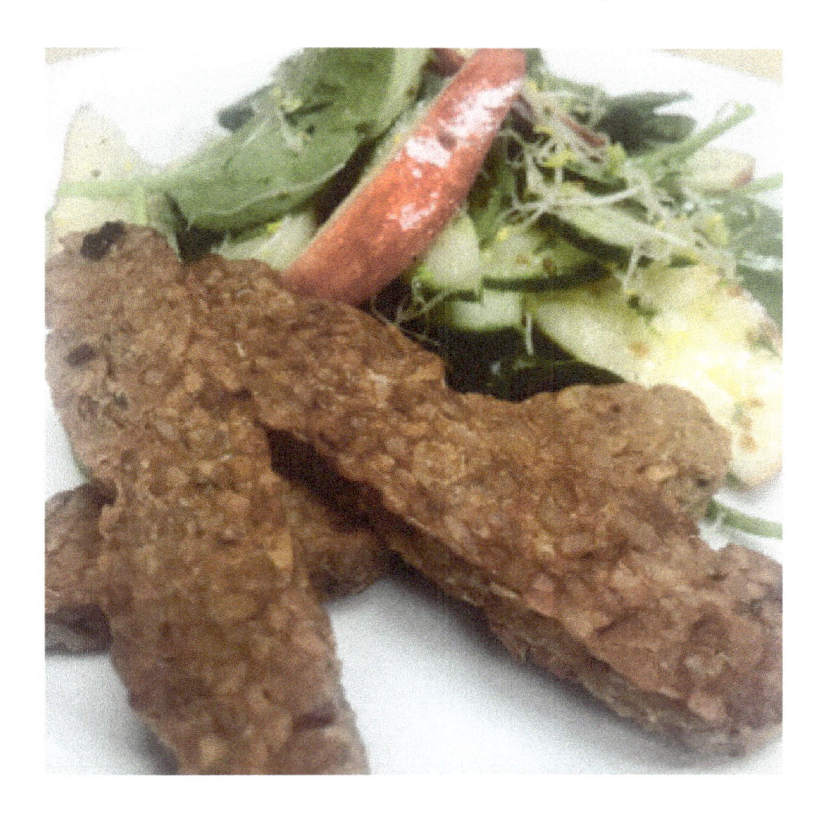

Sprouted seeds

You can buy sprouted alfalfa seeds and mung beans in many health food shops but it is easy to make your own sprouted seeds. Sprouted seeds provide a good source of protein and nutrients and are easier to digest than their unsprouted versions.

A mason jar works very well but any clean 1 litre jar will suffice. Use any edible seeds you like e.g. pumpkin, sunflower, sesame… Fill the bottom of the jar with your seeds (no more than one third full), rinse in cold water and then add enough lukewarm water to almost fill the jar. Cover the jar with a cloth and fix a rubber band.

Leave the seeds to soak overnight, rinse and drain them whilst still in the jar. Lay the jar on its side in a dark cupboard and continue to rinse and drain the seeds at least twice a day until fully sprouted – this can take up to 5 days. Drain and put in the fridge and use within a couple of days.

Sprouted broccoli seeds

Sprouted broccoli seeds are a great source of sulforaphane - a phytonutrient that has been shown to be cancer protective and excellent for liver detoxification. Sprouting your own broccoli seeds is very satisfying, easy and cheap. I bought 2 sprouting jars with the special lids quite cheaply from Amazon along with some organic sprouting broccoli seeds, which means I have one jar in the fridge and one sprouting at any one time. Add to salads and sandwiches every day.

Place 1-2 tablespoons of broccoli seeds in a clean wide mouth mason jar and cover with filtered water. Screw on the 'sprouting lid' and place the jar in a dark cupboard for 8 hours or covered by a tea towel in a warm place in the kitchen overnight.

After 8-12 hours drain off the water and rinse the seeds with fresh water, leave the jar at an angle to drain completely. Rinse and drain the sprouts twice a day, placing the jar back at an angle to drain thoroughly each time and keeping the jar covered. After a few days the seeds should have sprouted, continue to rinse and drain twice a day. Once the sprouts are 2cms long place the jar in sunlight so that the leaves turn a darker green.

Wait about 12 hours from the last rinse so that the sprouts are thoroughly drained and place the jar, with a regular air-tight lid, in the fridge ready to eat.

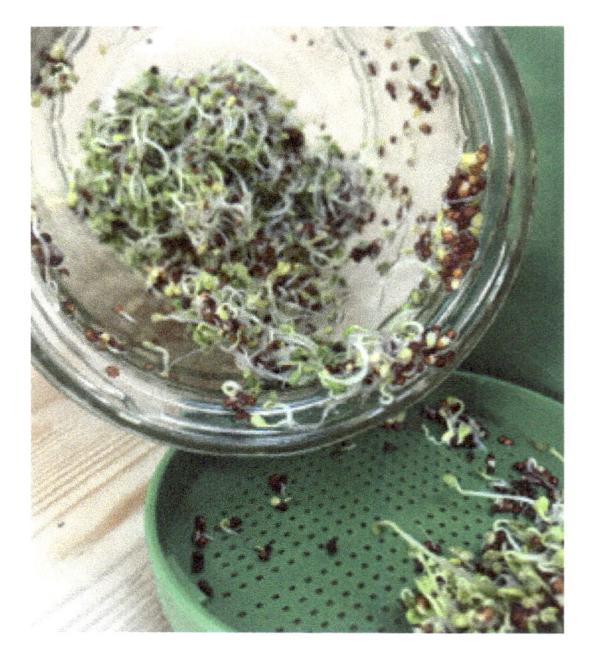

Tarka dahl

This recipe appeared in my last book but I had to include it again because it is the most perfect comfort food, it's easy to make and impresses guests every time. I always pray there is enough left for my lunch the next day.

Serves 6

250g red lentils, rinsed
3 tbsp olive oil
1 tbsp cumin seeds
1 small onion, peeled & chopped
3-4 green chillies, slit with seeds removed
20g fresh ginger, peeled and cut into thin strips
2 large cloves garlic, peeled

2 large cloves garlic, peeled
3-4 large tomatoes
sea salt
1 tsp turmeric
1 tsp garam masala
1 1/2 tsp ground coriander
handful fresh coriander leaves & stalks, chopped

Place the lentils and 800ml of water in a deep saucepan. Bring to the boil and skim off any froth. Cover and simmer for about 20 mins. adding more water if necessary.

Meanwhile, heat the oil in a small saucepan, add the cumin seeds and heat for a moment until fragrant. Add the onion, chillies and ginger and cook for about 10 mins until golden.

Purée the garlic and tomatoes in a blender, add to the onion mixture with the salt, spices and 100ml water. Cook for about 15 mins. over a moderate heat.

Stir the tomato mix into the cooked lentils, add more water if too thick. Bring to the boil, stir in the fresh coriander and serve.

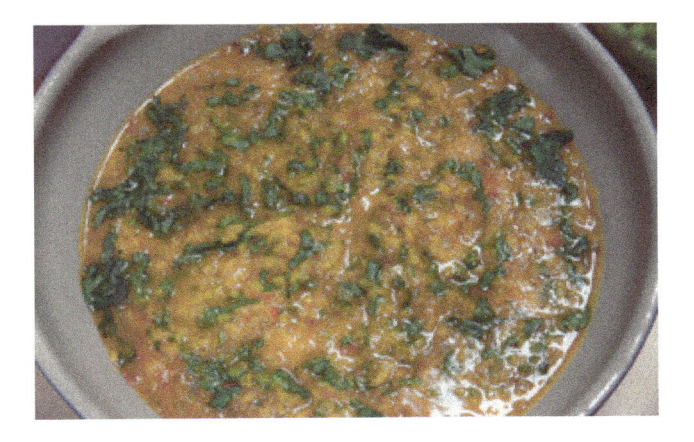

Cauliflower rice

Cauliflower is another cruciferous vegetables from the Brassica family (which includes cabbage, Brussel sprouts, kale, broccoli), these vegetables contain compounds which help to reduce the production of toxic intermediates during the detoxification process.

This recipe may seem a bit faddy but it is actually really good, and great if you are trying to reduce the amount of grains or starch in your diet.

Serves 4

half a large head of cauliflower
30g pine nuts
black pepper
juice 1/2 lemon
2 tsp tahini

Place the ingredients in a food processor and blend to a rice consistency.

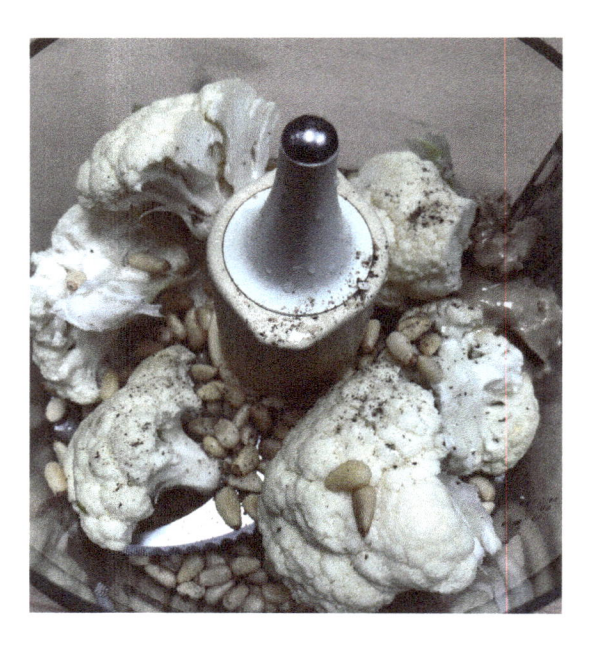

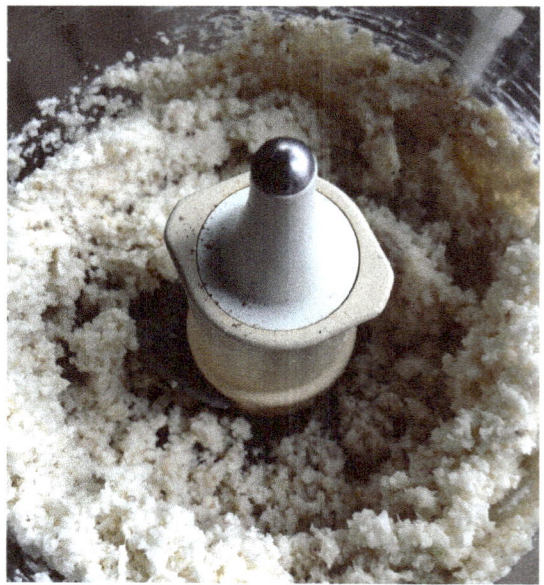

Whole roasted cauliflower

A bit trendy and probably a passing phase on the menu for many restaurants but certainly a good centre piece which will impress your friends and another way to replace the usual starch/grains that might otherwise accompany your meal. You could use the same dressing as for the roasted cauliflower salad - this one is pretty much the same with some chilli flakes added.

Serves 4

1 large cauliflower, green leaves removed and stalk cut so that the cauliflower sits upright in a casserole dish.

dressing:
1 tbsp wholegrain mustard
2 garlic cloves
2 tbsp apple cider vinegar
4 tbsp olive oil
1/2 tsp chilli flakes
sea salt & black pepper
fresh parsley, chopped

Pre heat the oven to 180°C.

Put all the dressing ingredients into a food processor and blitz to a smooth, creamy dressing. Place the cauliflower upright in a casserole dish and pour over the dressing, rub it into the whole cauliflower so it's completely coated.

Put the lid on the dish and roast the cauliflower in the oven for approx. half an hour, remove the lid and roast for another 5 minutes so that the cauliflower browns.

Transfer to a serving plate and garnish with chopped parsley.

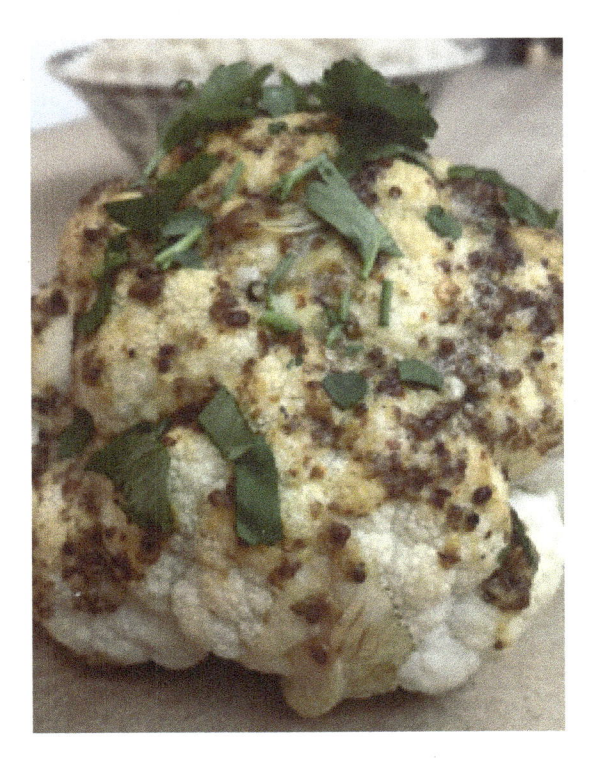

Ginger greens

This is a method for cooking any green vegetables and one which always goes down well with my family. I originally made this recipe with broccoli but now use it for green beans, pak choi, leeks – anything really ...

1 large head of broccoli, cut into florets or any green vegetables of your choice
fresh ginger, approx 3 tsp grated
1 tsp tamari soy sauce
1 tsp fish sauce
3 tbsp of water
1 tbsp olive oil/coconut oil
3 tsp sesame seeds
1 tsp sesame oil

Heat the oil in a heavy based frying pan or wok. Add the green vegetables and toss with a pair of tongs for a couple of minutes until they turn a darker shade of emerald green. Add the ginger and sesame seeds and continue to cook for a minute. Add the soy sauce, fish sauce, sesame oil and water and cover so that the greens continue to 'steam fry' for a minute until tender.

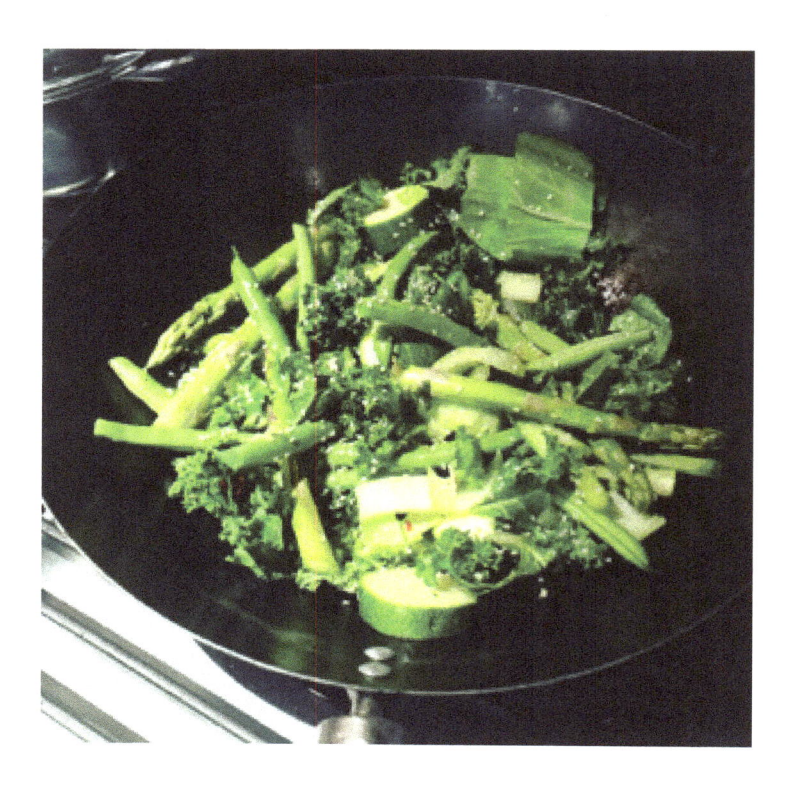

Ratatouille

Onion and garlic are a good source of the sulphur containing amino acids, which are important for detoxification in the liver. All these vegetables and herbs provide a generous amount of soluble fibre which helps the beneficial bacteria of your microbiome to thrive. A healthy microbiome will positively support your digestive, mental and immune health – all good reasons to eat more vegetables.

Serves 4

1 large red onion, sliced
4 tbsp olive oil
1 tsp sea salt
4 cloves garlic, finely chopped
250g cherry tomatoes, chopped
250g large tomatoes, chopped
2 400ml cans whole tomatoes
juice of half a lemon
2 tsp balsamic vinegar
1 large aubergine, sliced into thick rounds
2 red, yellow, or orange peppers, thickly sliced
3 courgettes, sliced lengthways
generous handful fresh basil leaves, chopped, plus more for garnish
a small handful fresh oregano leaves, removed from stem
5 sprigs of fresh thyme, chopped
cold-pressed olive oil for garnish

Add the onion to a large pan with 2 tbsp of the olive oil and salt. Cook gently for approx. 15 mins until the onion is soft and caramelized. Add the garlic, stir and after a minute add the canned tomatoes, breaking them up slightly with a wooden spoon. Add the fresh tomatoes, the lemon juice and the balsamic vinegar and leave to simmer gently (with a lid on) while you cook the other vegetables.

In another large pan heat 2 tbsp olive oil and gently cook the aubergine, courgette and pepper for approx. 5 mins until tender. (Alternatively you could brush these vegetables with olive oil and grill/griddle them on both sides)

Add the vegetables to the tomato mix with the herbs and season with sea salt and freshly ground black pepper, continue to simmer for another 5 minutes. To add more protein you may like to stir in some cooked Puy lentils – you can buy these ready cooked (Merchant Gourmet) from large supermarkets. Serve with an extra drizzle of olive oil and some fresh basil leaves.

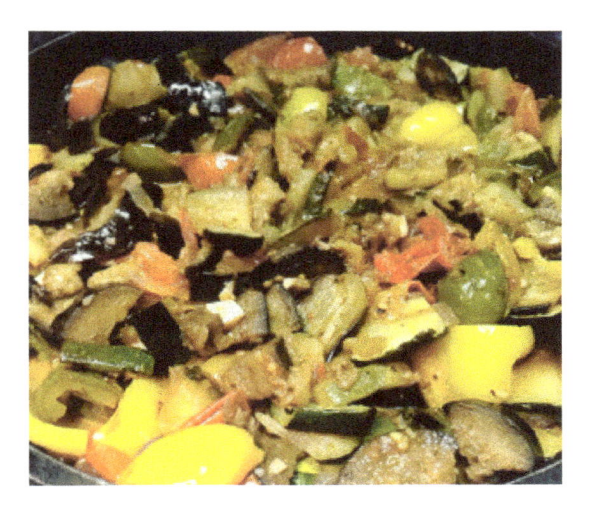

Sweet potato wedges

Preheat the oven to 180°C. Cut the sweet potatoes (1 medium potato per head) into thick wedges, place on a baking tray. Drizzle with some olive oil or melted coconut oil and sprinkle with sea salt. Bake in the oven for approx. 25 mins until tender.

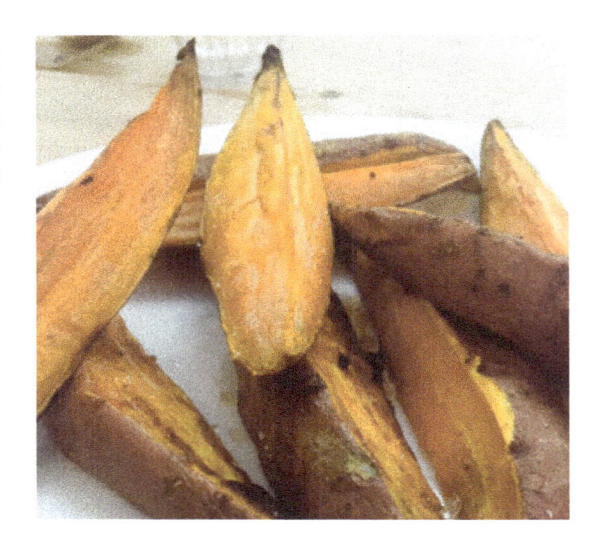

Roasted veggies

I like to roast root vegetables, you can choose from white/sweet potatoes, pumpkin, butternut squash, parsnips, carrots and beetroot along with onions and garlic.

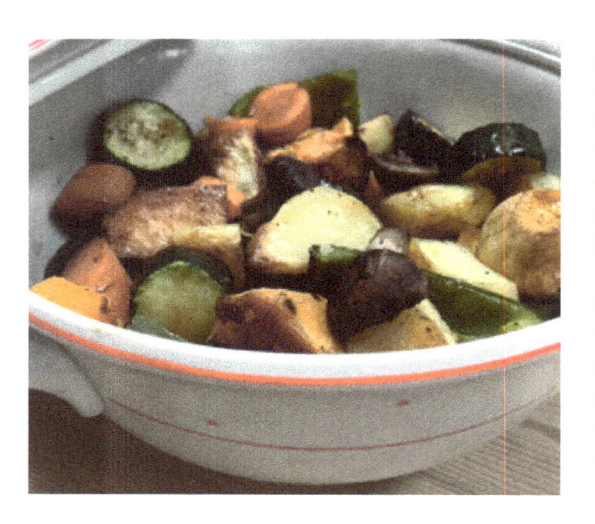

Preheat the oven to 180°C. Cut all the vegetables into roughly equal sized pieces and, leaving the garlic cloves unpeeled, arrange all the vegetables in a single layer on a large baking tray/dish. Drizzle with olive oil or melted coconut oil and sprinkle with sea salt and freshly ground black pepper. Add a few sprigs of rosemary.

Roast in the oven for approx. 30 mins until tender. 15 mins before the end of the cooking time you could add chopped red peppers, courgette and mushrooms. The garlic can be squeezed out of each clove once cooking is complete.

Fresh spring rolls

I like to serve these fresh tasting spring rolls with drinks when friends come over but they would also be great with a big salad as a lunch. I sometimes include thin strips of marinated tofu or I make a tiny single egg omelette and use thin 'egg strips' in the rolls. If you eat fish then you can experiment with prawns and smoked salmon, the variations are endless...

Serves 4

8 rice wrappers (from Thai supermarket or health food shop)
1 chopped & deseeded chilli
1 small piece of ginger, grated
2 garlic cloves, finely chopped
2 tsp tamari soy sauce
juice of 1 lime
100g vermicelli rice noodles

1 carrot, cut into thin strips
2 spring onions, cut into strips
1/4 chinese leaf lettuce, finely chopped
mint leaves, large handful
basil & coriander leaves, large handful (Thai basil works really well)
half a yellow and half a red pepper, sliced into thick strips

Pour boiling water over the rice noodles in a bowl and leave to stand for 3 mins. (or as instructed on packet) then drain and run under cold water to prevent further cooking. Combine the chilli, soy sauce, lime juice, ginger and garlic in a large bowl and add the noodles, giving them a stir so that they soak up the flavours.

In a large shallow dish soak a rice paper wrapper in warm water for about 20 seconds.
Carefully lie the rice wrapper flat on a damp tea towel and then place a tbsp of the noodles and a little of each of the vegetables and herbs onto the middle of the wrapper. Fold into a packet/parcel. Keep fresh in the fridge covered with a damp tea towel until ready to eat.

Serve with some tamari soy sauce or sweet chilli dipping sauce.

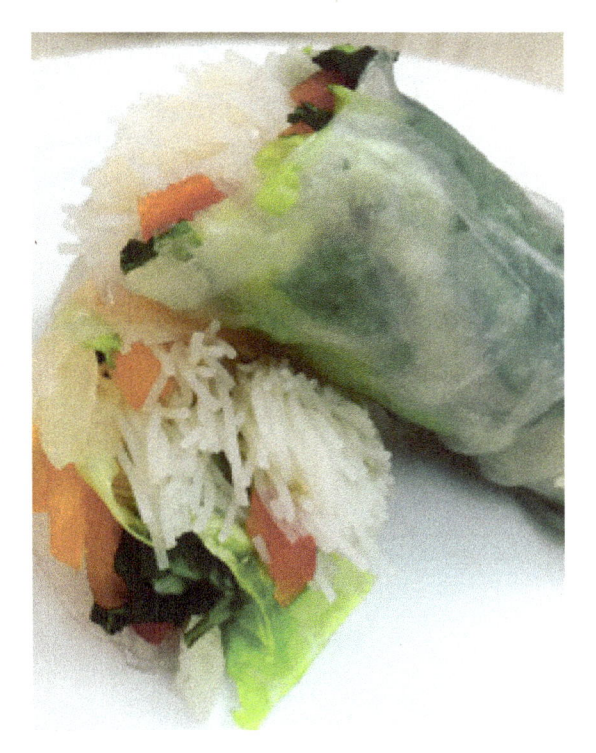

Cashew cheese

I wasn't sure where to put this recipe, not really a side dish but a useful little recipe if you are vegan and need something quick to go on top of a cracker, makes a change from the usual hummus.

This recipe uses nutritional yeast flakes which add a cheesy flavour and are a good source of B vitamins including B12 which is often deficient in vegan diets.

Serves 4

250g cashews
2 tbsp Engevita nutritional yeast flakes
1 lemon, juiced
half tsp sea salt
1 tbsp water
1 tbsp chives/dill, chopped

Soak the cashews in a bowl overnight by covering them with plenty of water. Rinse and drain and add to the food processor with the Engevita yeast flakes, lemon juice, salt and water. Blend to a smooth paste – this may take about 5 minutes, and you will need to scrape the mixture down from the sides of the processor a few times. Add the chopped chives or dill and keep in the fridge.

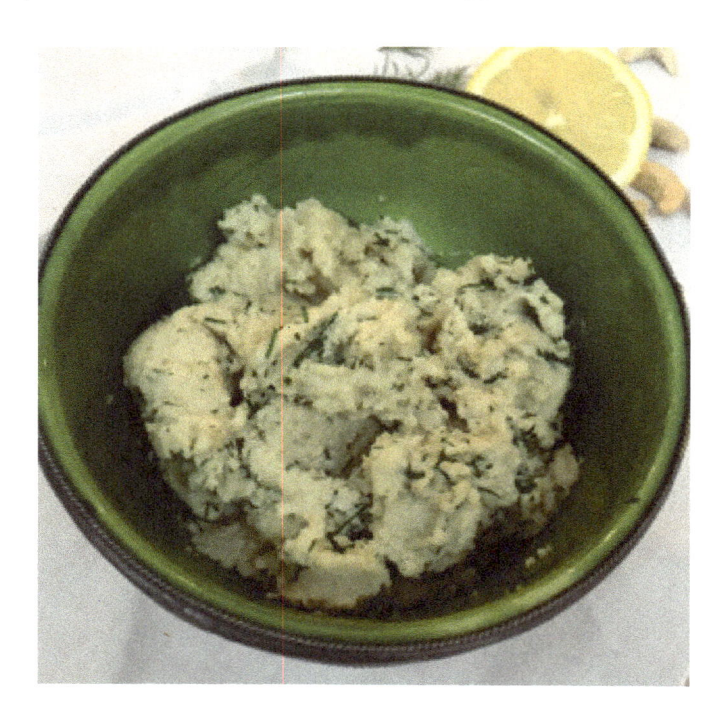

Salads

It's hard to choose which salads to include in this chapter as the variations are endless and to be honest, I usually make things up as I go along depending on what ingredients I have in the fridge, you might notice that I absolutely love feta and add it to salads whenever I can. The secret to a good salad is the dressing – this is what really brings it alive. The salads I have chosen have all featured and have been popular at my cookery workshops.

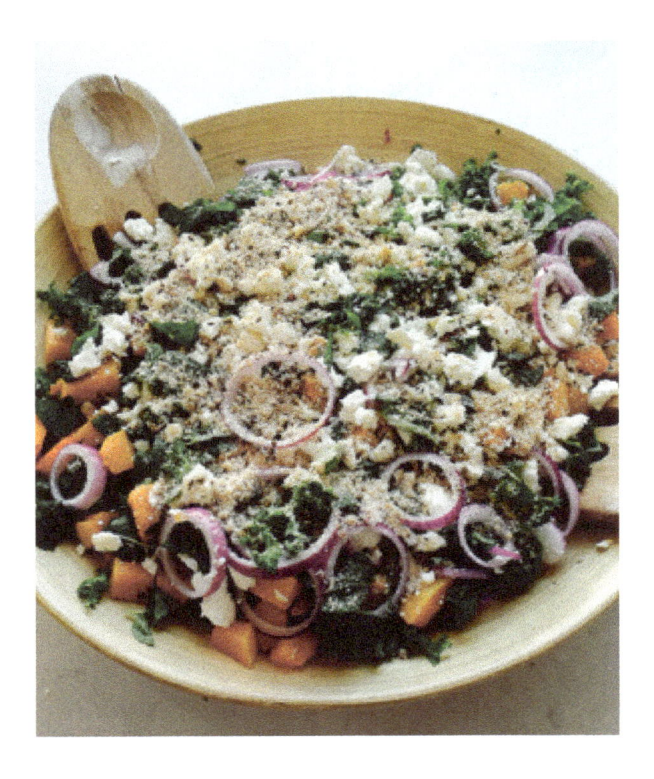

Winter slaw

This recipe keeps for a few days so can be made up in advance over the weekend.

1 tbsp pumpkin seeds
1/4 white cabbage, shredded
1 baby gem lettuce, finely sliced
6 radishes, finely sliced
1 small red onion, finely sliced
1 large carrot, sliced into matchsticks
half red chilli, finely sliced
2 tbsp chopped fresh mint
1 tbsp chopped fresh coriander

dressing:
1 tsp cumin seeds
1/2 tsp Dijon mustard
1 garlic clove, finely chopped
large pinch sea salt
2 tsp red wine vinegar
juice of half a lime
150ml extra virgin olive oil
1 tbsp natural yoghurt /soya or nut yoghurt

Dry roast the cumin seeds in a heavy based frying pan for a minute and then grind to a powder with a pestle and mortar.

In a small bowl mix the mustard, garlic, cumin, salt, vinegar and lime juice. Gradually whisk in the olive oil. Stir in the yoghurt.

Dry roast the pumpkin seeds in a heavy based pan for a minute until the skins are popping. In a large bowl mix all the slaw ingredients. Toss the slaw with the dressing just before serving – you may like to use a little less dressing so taste as you add to get desired amount.

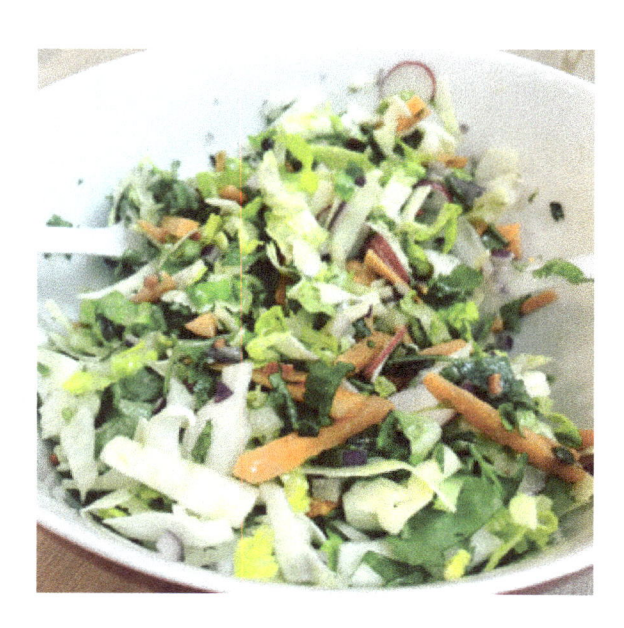

Roasted butternut squash salad with Dukkah

It may seem like a bit of a hassle to make this Dukkah topping but it lasts in a glass jar in the fridge for at least a month and will bring any salad or vegetablesgie dish to life. Dukkah is a classic Egyptian condiment.

1 large butternut squash, peeled & cubed
sea salt & black pepper
1 bunch kale, chopped (150g)
cold pressed olive oil
juice of half a lemon
200g feta
handful fresh mint leaves, chopped
1 small red onion, cut into fine rings

dukkah:
1 tbsp coriander seeds
1½ tbsp cumin seeds
1 tbsp whole black peppercorns
140g raw hazelnuts (skinned)
70g sesame seeds

Roast the butternut squash in the oven with a little coconut oil or brushed with olive oil for approx. 30 mins. Remove any tough pieces of kale and in a large bowl drizzle over the olive oil, a little salt, black pepper and the lemon juice. Using your hands rub the kale together for a couple of minutes.

Top the kale with the butternut squash and crumble over the feta. Garnish with chopped mint, red onion, and a dusting of Dukkah.

For the dukkah, toast the coriander and cumin seeds in a dry pan for a couple of minutes. Grind the seeds with the peppercorns in a pestle and mortar. Toast the hazelnuts and sesame seeds in the same pan for a few minutes and put in the food processor – pulse to a chunky texture. Add the ground coriander mix to the nut mix with a little sea salt and combine.

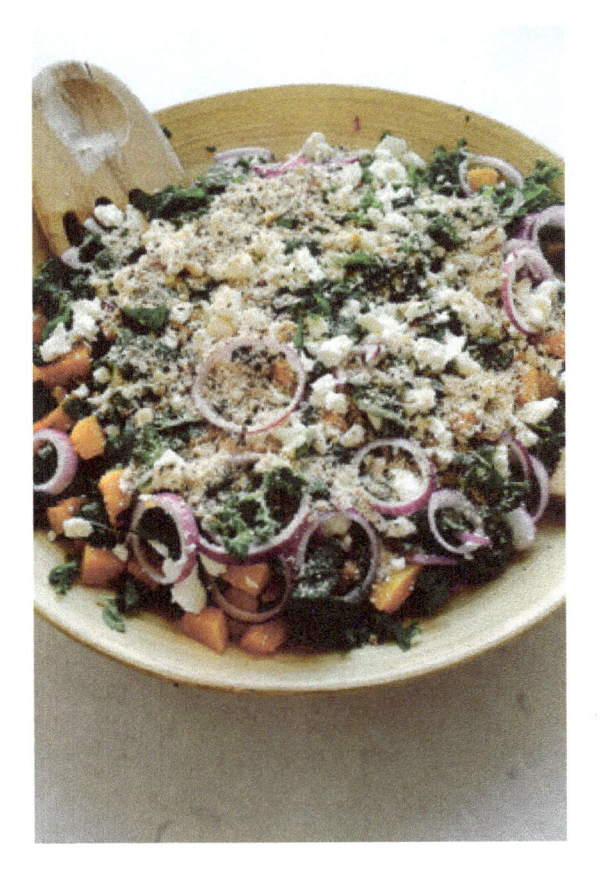

Avocado and tomato salad

This is from my first book, inspired by Antony Worrall Thompson and very popular with friends and family (that's you Zara!)

flesh of 2 ripe Hass avocados, cubed
1 red onion, diced finely
1 large bunch of washed and dried coriander, chopped
1 punnet of sweet cherry tomatoes, halved
juice of 1 lime
black pepper & sea salt

Combine all of the ingredients in a large bowl
– simple.

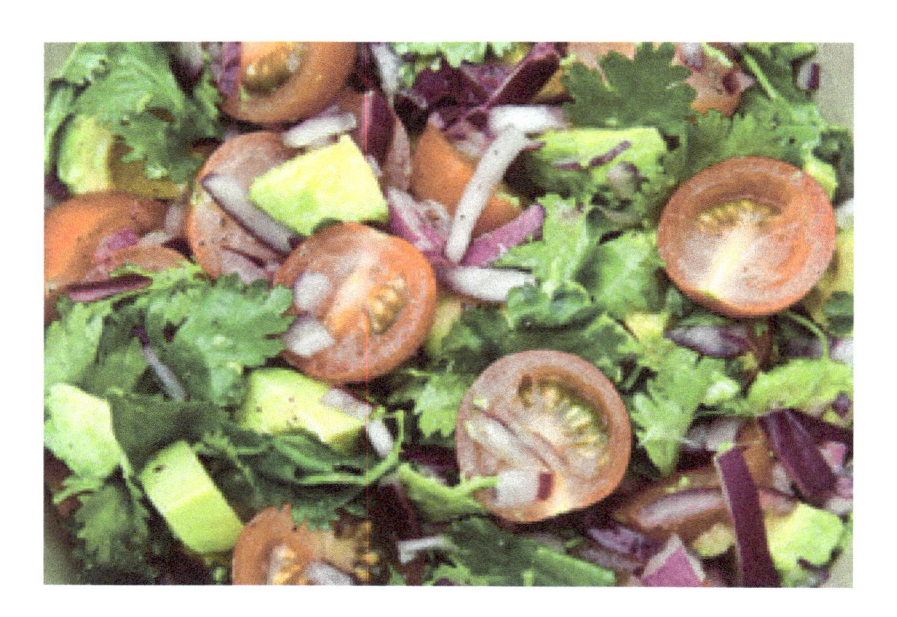

Spinach salad with sesame and tamari

Spinach is such a versatile vegetable, I love to use it raw in salads and this recipe is fabulous alongside any meal.

Serves 4

1 small shallot, finely chopped
1 small piece of ginger, peeled and finely chopped or grated
2 tbsp rice wine vinegar
1 tbsp tamari soy sauce

1 tbsp toasted sesame oil
200g baby spinach leaves, washed
1 avocado, sliced
2 spring onions, cut into fine rings
2 tbsp toasted sesame seeds

Mix the shallot, ginger, vinegar, tamari and sesame oil with 1 tsp sea salt and set aside. Put the spinach leaves into a large bowl and add the dressing. Add the avocado, spring onion and sesame seeds and serve immediately before the spinach starts to wilt.

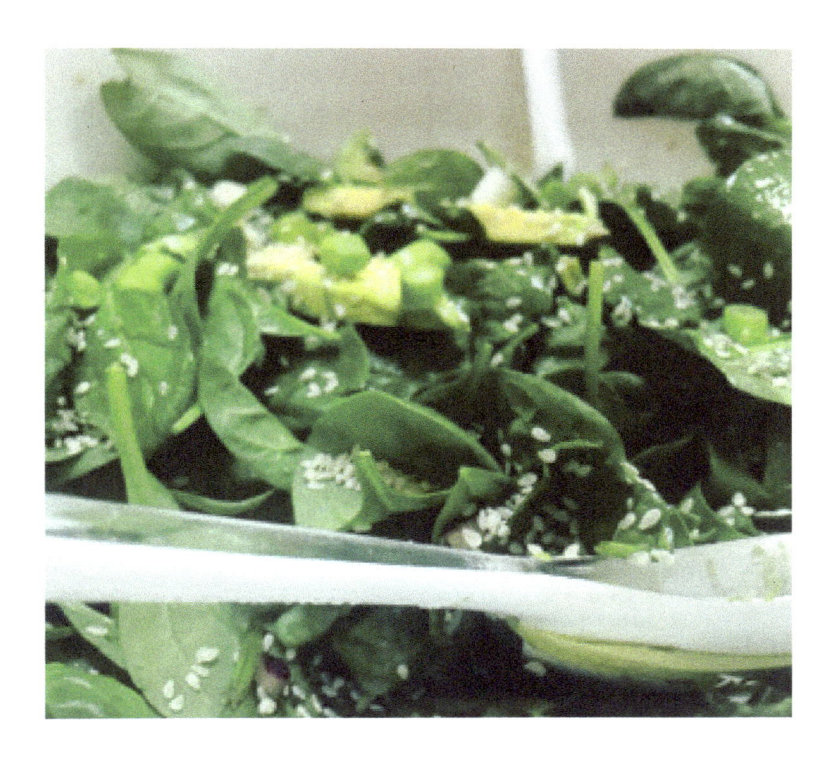

Nigella's avocado and red onion salad

Nigella comes up with some great salads and I love this one – it makes a great starter as the colours are really vibrant and is it quick and easy to prepare before your guests arrive.

Serves 4

half a small red onion
red wine vinegar
1 ripe avocado
50g feta

black onion seeds
pomegranate seeds
extra virgin olive oil
sea salt and black pepper

Slice the onion into fine rings and place in a small bowl, cover with red wine vinegar. Leave for 30 minutes.

Meanwhile, slice the avocado flesh into strips and arrange on a plate, crumble over the feta, sprinkle with black onion and pomegranate seeds. Drain the onion rings and add to salad.

Drizzle with olive oil and season with sea salt and black pepper.

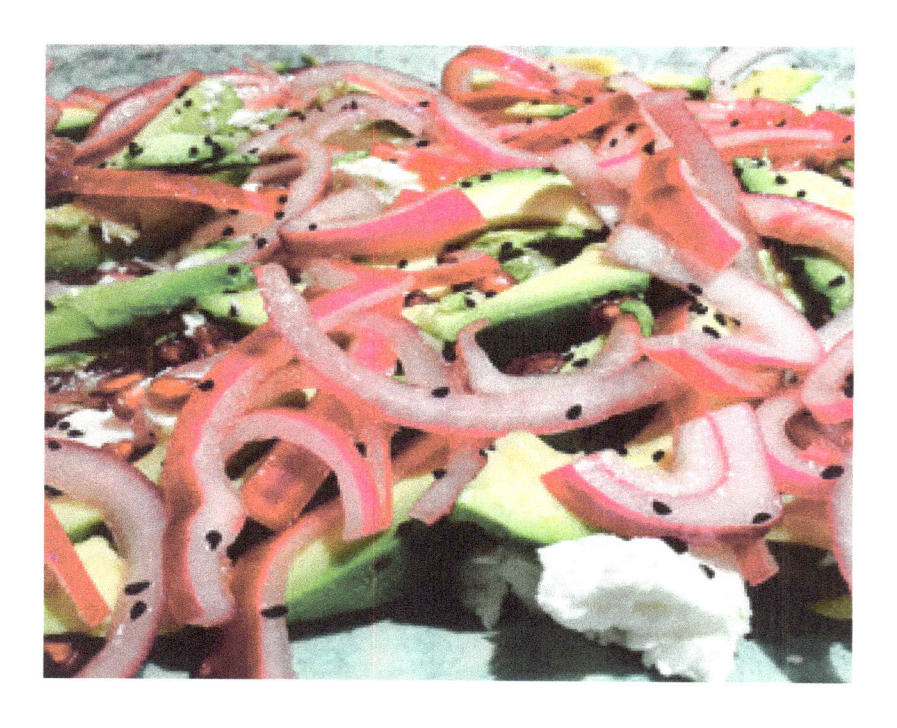

Japanese salad

I love this salad and especially love the dressing which tastes wonderfully authentic – the miso and umeboshi purée are the secret ingredients. I like to add tofu, stir fried in a little olive or coconut oil, but also like to eat the salad with fish or sushi. I buy all my Japanese ingredients from my local Windfall Natural health shop as they stock the brand Clearspring which has fantastic products.

Serves 2

1 large carrot
1 courgette
handful green beans, thinly sliced
small handful Thai basil leaves, ripped
handful coriander leaves
handful alfalfa/bean sprouts
seeds from half pomegranate
50g raw cashews

dressing:
1 tbsp white miso paste
2 tbsp mirin
1 tsp sesame oil
2 tsp umeboshi plum puree
1 pack sushi ginger (50g drained weight)
2 tsp rice wine vinegar
1 tbsp lime juice
2 tbsp water

Whizz the dressing ingredients in a blender until smooth.

Use a spiralizer to make the carrot and courgette into spirals in a large bowl and mix. Mix in the beans, herbs, sprouts and pomegranate seeds. Add some of the dressing to the salad and toss gently, adding more dressing to taste.

Scatter on the cashews before serving. (Dressing will last in fridge for a few days).

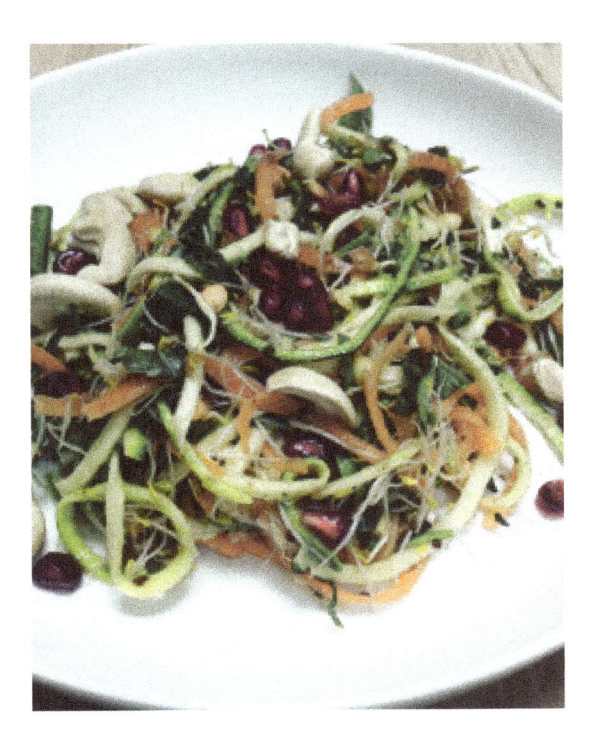

Chargrilled cauliflower salad

This is the perfect Summer salad as you can griddle the cauliflower on the bbq – just as good in Winter though.

Serves 4

2 tbsp capers, drained
1 tbsp wholegrain mustard
2 garlic cloves
2 tbsp apple cider vinegar
100ml extra virgin olive oil

1 cauliflower head, cut into small florets
1 tbsp chopped dill
50g spinach leaves
20 cherry tomatoes, halved
sea salt and black pepper

In a food processor blend the capers, mustard, garlic, vinegar and some sea salt and black pepper. Gradually add 50ml of the oil to make a thick and creamy dressing. Add the cauliflower florets to a large pan of boiling water and simmer for 3 mins. Drain and run under cold water. Leave to dry and then place in a bowl with the remaining oil, toss well.

Heat a ridged griddle pan/bbq and then grill the cauliflower in batches.

In a serving bowl add some of the dressing to the hot charred cauliflower florets along with the spinach and tomatoes. Stir and season/add more dressing if necessary.

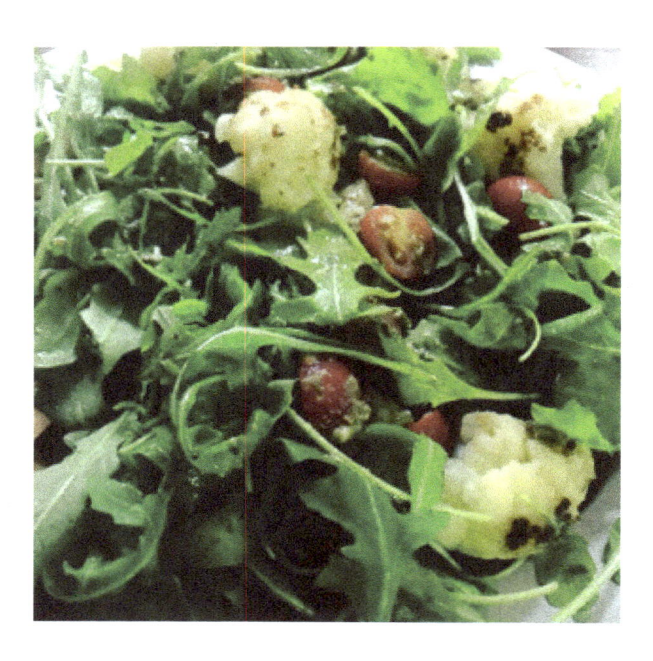

Courgetti with feta and herb pistachio pesto

Serves 4

200g feta
1 unwaxed lemon, zested.
a good pinch of chilli flakes
60g shelled pistachios

extra virgin olive oil
1 small bunch of fresh mint
small bunch of fresh basil
4 large courgettes

Toast the pistachios in the oven for 3-5 minutes.

Put the toasted pistachios into the food processor, adding the leaves from the basil and mint, add the juice of half a lemon and a good pinch of sea salt. Add 4 tablespoons of olive oil and a tablespoon of cold water and pulse until you have a textured pesto and transfer to a bowl.

Use a julienne peeler or a spiralizer to make courgetti/courgette noodles. Toss the pesto through the courgetti.

Crumble over the feta, adding lemon zest and chilli flakes.

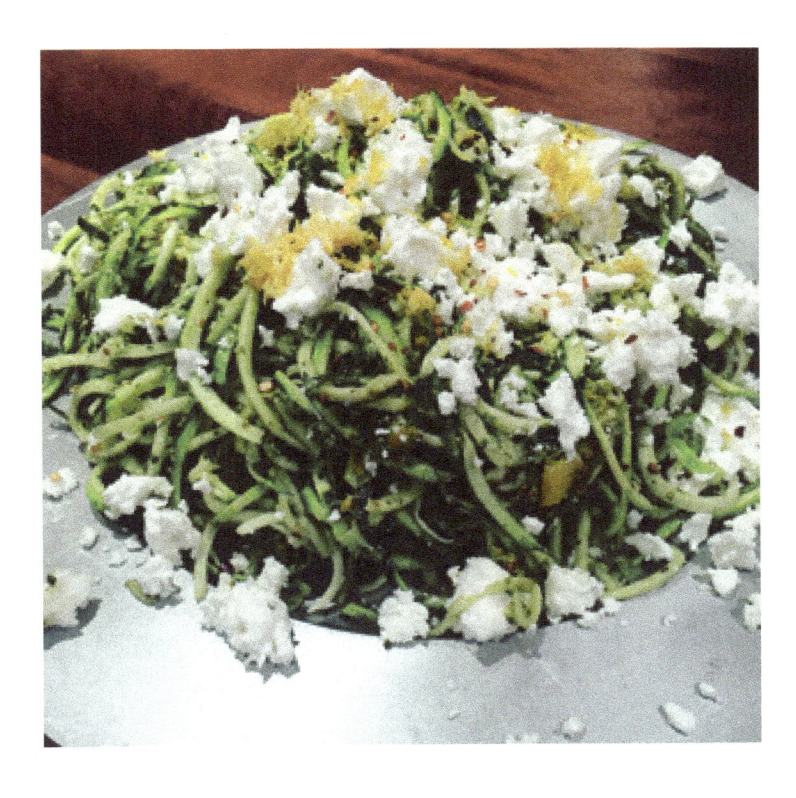

Chickpea and feta salad

This salad, another Feed Your Health classic, is packed with ingredients to support immune health; it uses plenty of fresh herbs, lemon juice and chilli which all contain good levels of vitamin C.

Serves 4

400g tinned chickpeas
3 tbsp olive oil
1 large red onion
5 garlic cloves
1 red chilli

200g crumbled feta cheese
4 spring onions, chopped
large handful chopped coriander
large handful chopped flat leaf parsley
juice of 1 lemon

Rinse the chickpeas and put them in a bowl. Heat the olive oil and sauté the red onion gently until it is softened. Add the garlic and chilli and cook for another minute, leave to cool.

Add the feta, spring onion, coriander, parsley and lemon juice to the chickpeas and season with black pepper and a little sea salt. Add the cooled garlic, chilli and onion and mix well.

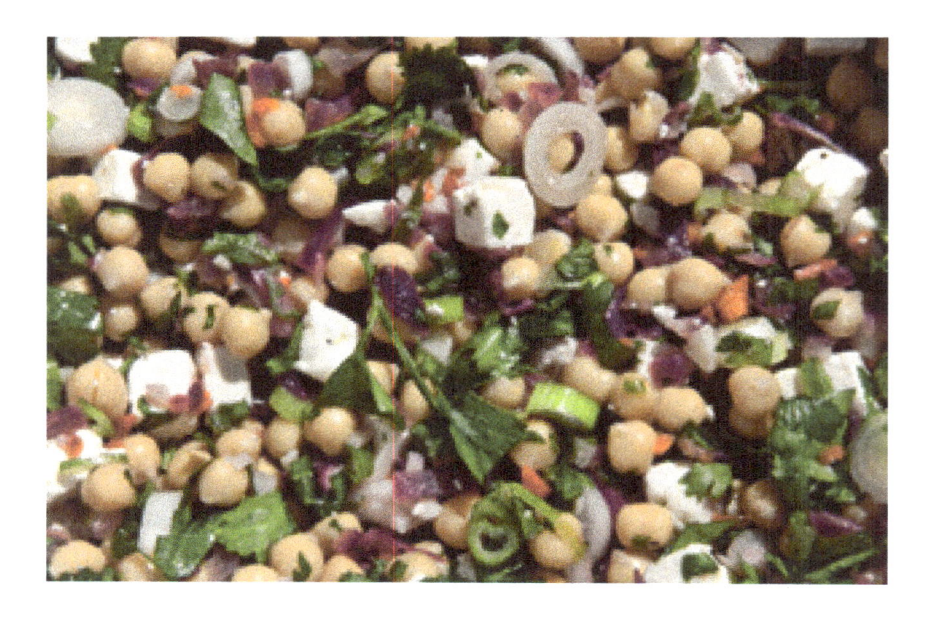

Pomegranate, chickpea and mint salad

Years ago I went to a cooking demo hosted by Nanette Newman and this is from her book 'Eating In', I included it in my last book and have to put it in again as everyone loves it.

Serves 4

4 spring onions, finely sliced
1 garlic clove, finely sliced
a small handful of mint leaves, roughly shredded
olive oil

I can of rinsed and drained chickpeas
grated zest and juice of 1 lemon
seeds of 1 pomegranate
sea salt & ground black pepper

Combine all of the ingredients for a refreshing and delicious salad.

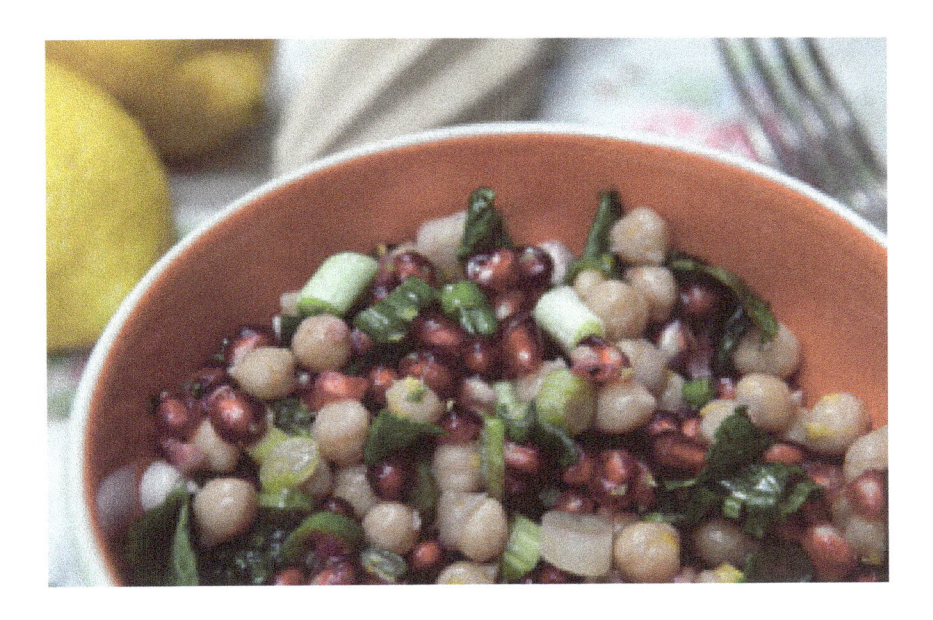

Coconut and lime salad

I found this salad in a magazine I was reading on a flight and just knew I would love it – the coconut and lime make it taste so fresh, it has a Summery, clean taste which works really well with any main course but I love to serve it alongside the Thai Laksa.

Serves 4

1 large bunch of flat leaf parsley, finely chopped
1 bunch of mint leaves, finely chopped
100g freshly grated coconut
(I use my food processor for this)
2 limes, juiced

1 small red onion, thinly sliced
large handful cherry tomatoes, chopped
2 spring onions, finely chopped
2 celery sticks, finely sliced
seeds from 1 pomegranate

Place the grated coconut in a bowl and season with the lime juice, sea salt and black pepper. Add the rest of the ingredients and mix well.

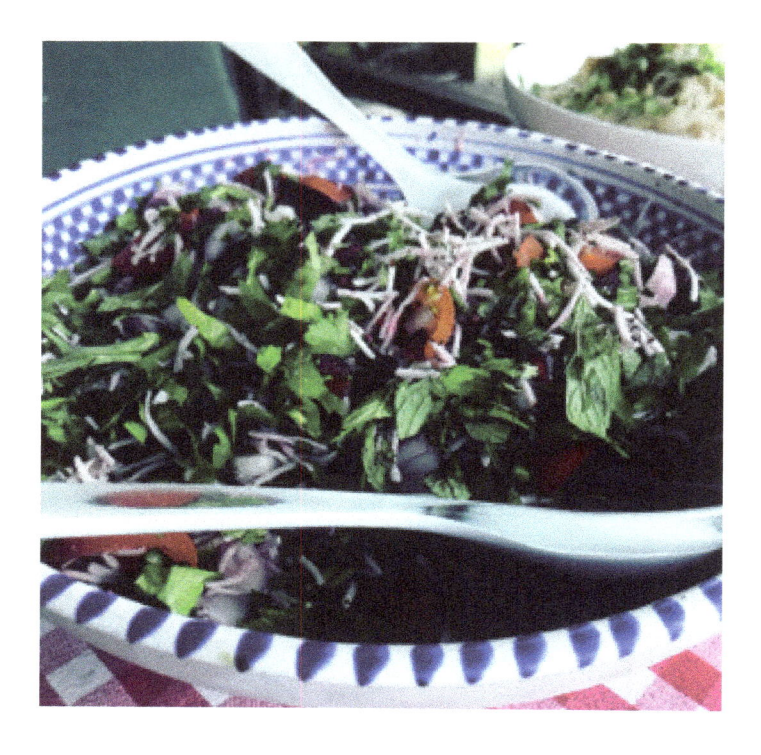

Mains

All of these main course recipes have been tried and tested at my Cookery Workshops. I love these events, especially at the end when we all sit down to enjoy the food we've created – that part never feels like work.

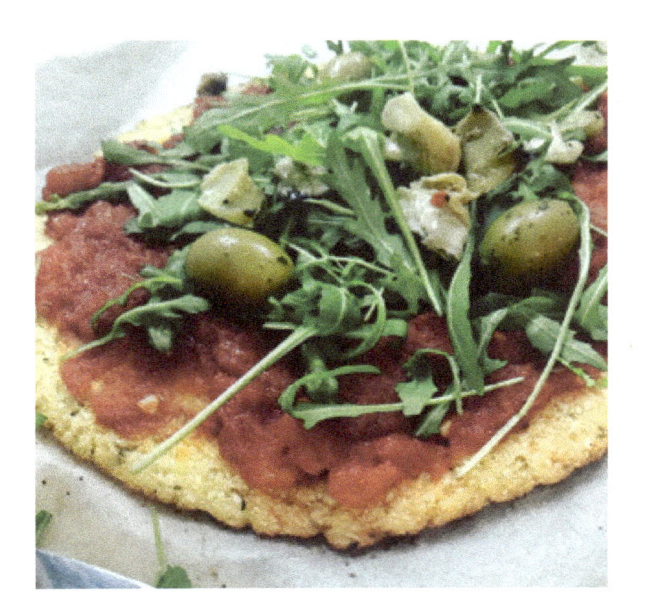

Fishy Mains

Moroccan fish tagine with potatoes, tomatoes, peppers & olives

When I first made this for the family I got the thumbs up which I knew was a good sign as they are pretty harsh critics – I then made it at a cookery workshop in Chobham and there was actually a shortage of cod in the area for a few days after the event as the supermarkets were stripped of supplies! It may seem a bit complicated but if you are making this for friends you can do most of it in advance so that when your guests arrive it is just an assembly project.

Serves 4

4 haddock/cod steaks, or any thick white fish fillets (skinless & boneless)
20 small waxy new potatoes, (Charlotte are good)
3 tbsp olive oil
4 garlic cloves, thinly sliced
15 cherry tomatoes, halved
4 green peppers, roasted and skinned, seeded and sliced into strips
1 handful black, oily olives
100ml water
sea salt, black pepper

charmoula marinade:
2 garlic cloves
1 level tsp sea salt
2 tsp freshly ground cumin
juice of 1 lemon
half tbsp red wine vinegar
1 tsp paprika
1 small bunch of fresh coriander, roughly chopped
1 tbsp olive oil

To make the charmoula, pound the garlic and salt to a paste in a pestle and mortar, add the cumin, lemon juice, vinegar, paprika, coriander and oil. Rub two thirds of the marinade into the fish and set aside in the fridge for 20 mins.

Boil the potatoes in salted water until just tender, then drain.

In a heavy pan sauté the garlic in 2 tbsp of olive oil, add the tomatoes and cook for a couple of mins., add the peppers and remaining charmoula.

In a 25cm tagine or frying pan with a lid, spread the potatoes evenly over the bottom. Scatter three quarters of the tomato mixture over the potatoes, then place the marinated fish on top. Dab a little of the remaining tomato mix and a few olives on top of each piece of fish. Add the water and drizzle on the last tbsp olive oil, put the lid on and steam over a high heat for 10 mins. Serve with a green salad.

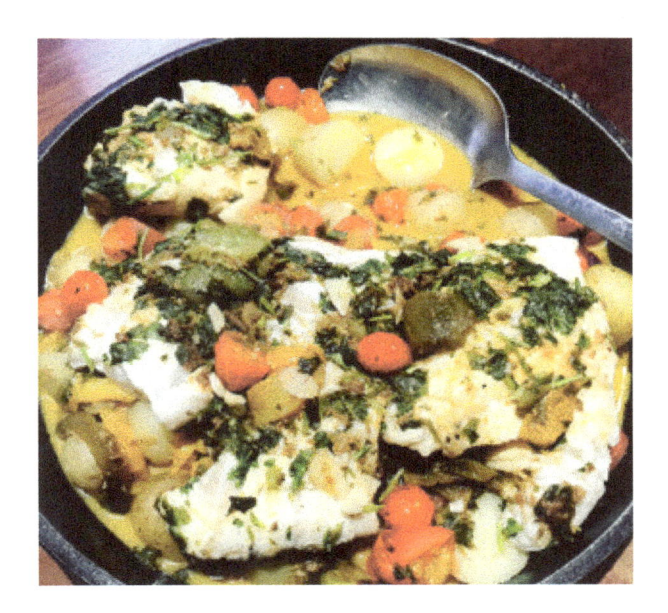

Miso salmon with radish and courgette salad

This is a dish that is perfect for everyone but its winning combination of omega 3 essential fats and soy phytoestrogens means it is also a good recipe for female hormone balance.

Serves 4

2 tbsp sesame seeds
2 tbsp sweet miso paste
1 tsp tamari
2 cloves of garlic, peeled and crushed
4 salmon fillets
1 small bunch of coriander, chopped
1 courgette, spirilized
50g radishes, finely sliced

dressing:
1 tbsp freshly grated ginger
half tsp tamari
1 tsp sesame oil
1 lime, juiced

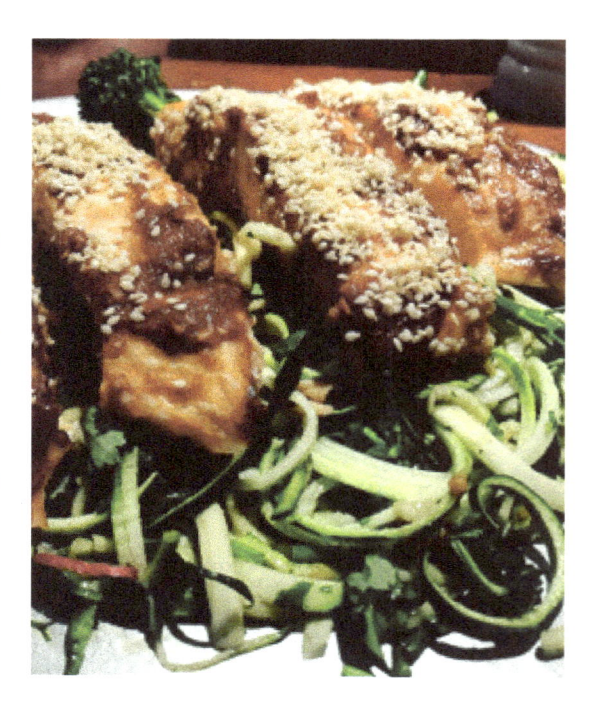

Preheat oven to 180°C.

Toast the sesame seeds in a dry pan over a medium heat, shaking to prevent burning. Set aside.

Mix the miso with the tamari and garlic and rub into the salmon fillets, place the fillets on a baking tray. Roast the salmon in the oven for 10-12 minutes until cooked through.

Mix all the dressing ingredients together and set aside.

Combine the coriander, courgette and radishes in a large bowl. Massage the dressing into the vegetables.

Arrange the vegetables on a serving plate, place the salmon on top and sprinkle with the toasted sesame seeds.

Fish and salsa parcels

Serves 4

4 chunky white fish fillets (cod or haddock)
12 cherry tomatoes, quartered
4 spring onions, trimmed & chopped
2 tbsp chopped coriander
1 tsp chopped chilli

3 tbsp olive oil
1 tbsp lemon juice
pinch sea salt
freshly ground black pepper
juice of 1 lime

Place the fish on the paper and sprinkle with salt and pepper. Combine all the salsa ingredients and divide evenly over the 4 fish fillets.

Seal the parcels and bake for 15 minutes. Drizzle with more lime juice before serving.

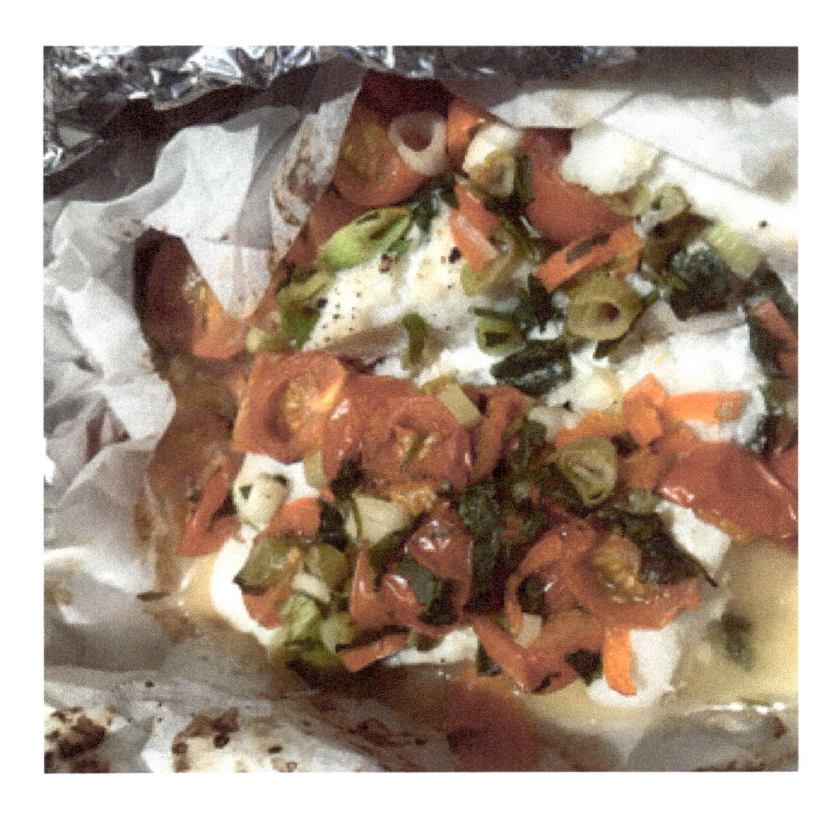

Prawn and tofu pad Thai

Serves 4

250g Thai flat rice noodles
200g tofu, cut into small pieces (2cm)
small pinch cayenne pepper
2 tsp tamarind paste
3 tbsp fish sauce
2 tsp coconut palm sugar
1 garlic clove, finely chopped
4 spring onions, cut into thin stips

2 tbsp olive oil
2 eggs, beaten
200g pack large cooked prawns
150g beansprouts
handful toasted cashews, chopped
handful coriander leaves to serve
lime wedges to serve

In a large shallow dish spread out the noodles and cover with boiling water. Leave to stand until the noodles are soft (follow packet directions), drain and then rinse under cold running water to stop further cooking. Set aside.

Heat 2 tbsp olive oil in a wok and stir fry the tofu pieces until they are golden, remove and set aside.

Mix the tamarind paste, cayenne pepper, fish sauce and sugar in a small bowl.

Pour another 2 tbsp of olive oil into the wok and swirl around to cover the base and sides. Add the garlic and spring onions, keep these moving with tongs for half a minute until they start to soften.

Push the vegetables to the side of the wok, add the egg to the middle of the wok and stir for 30 secs until it starts to set and looks like a broken omelette.

Add the prawns, tofu and beansprouts, then the noodles, then pour over the fish sauce mixture.

Toss everything together to heat through. Serve onto 4 plates or 1 large serving plate and add cashews and a sprinkling of coriander, finish with a wedges of lime on the side.

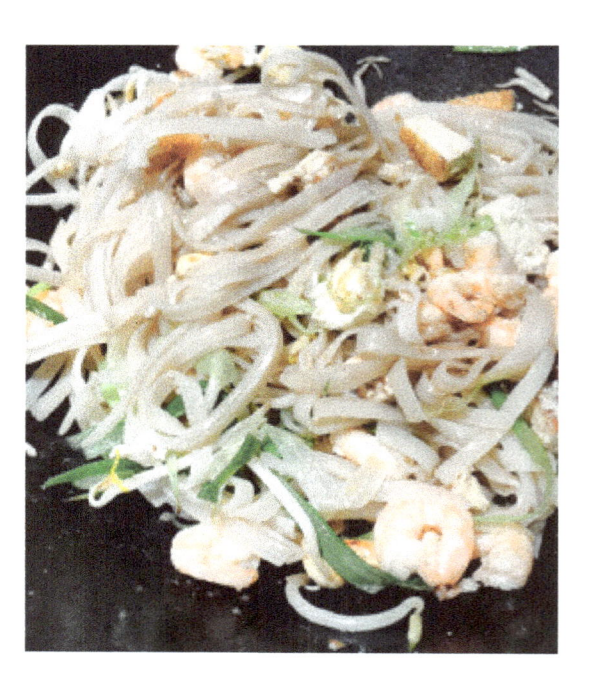

Salmon burgers with a fruity salsa

Makes 6 burgers

for the salsa:
half a cucumber, diced
half a mango, diced
one third pineapple, diced
half red chili, finely chopped
half small red onion, finely chopped
1 small bunch of coriander, chopped
1 small bunch of mint leaves, chopped
juice of 1 lime
sea salt

for the burgers:
750g salmon fillets, skinless
1 heaped tbsp sushi ginger
half small red onion, chopped
1 small bunch of coriander
2 tsp tamari soy sauce
2 tsp toasted sesame oil
half tsp sea salt
black pepper
olive oil

Combine salsa ingredients in a bowl and set aside.

Place the salmon on a plate and put it in the freezer for 15 mins along with the bowl and blade from the food processor.

Meanwhile prepare the rest of the burger ingredients. Blitz the cold salmon until roughly minced, (pulse for a couple of seconds about 6 times – the cold temperature prevents the salmon from turning to paste!)

Place the salmon in a large mixing bowl and use the processor to blitz the ginger, onion, coriander, tamari, sesame oil, salt and pepper. Add this to the salmon and combine with a spatula. Form the mixture into burgers. Put the burgers in the fridge to marinate for an hour, time permitting.

Heat a grill pan over a medium/high heat. Drizzle the burgers with a little olive oil and cook for about 5 minutes each side until browned. Serve with the salsa.

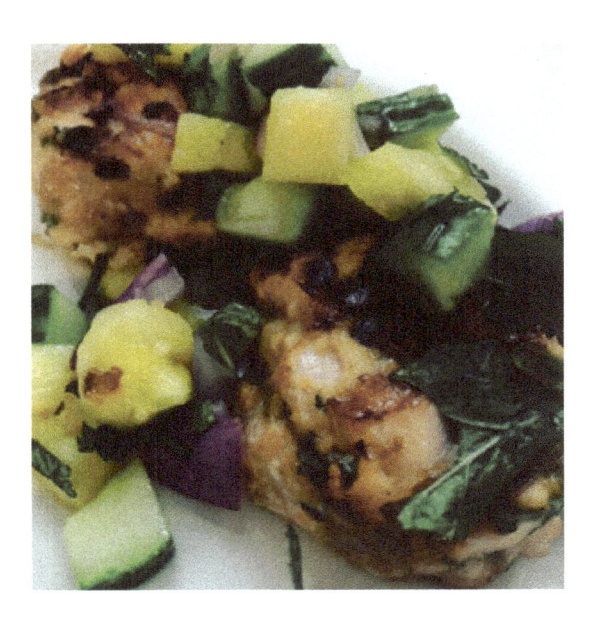

Mexican spicy salmon

Serves 4

zest and juice of 1 lime
1 1/2 tsp Chipotles en adobo
(or 1 red chilli, chopped finely)
1 tbsp maple syrup
sea salt
4 fillets of salmon

Preheat oven to 200°C.

Whisk together the lime zest and juice, the Chipotles en adobe and maple syrup along with a pinch of salt. Line a baking tray with parchment paper, place the salmon on the paper and pour the mixture over the salmon. Bake in the oven for about 15 mins. or until the salmon is just cooked through (timing depends on the thickness of the fillet).

Serve with a guacomole.

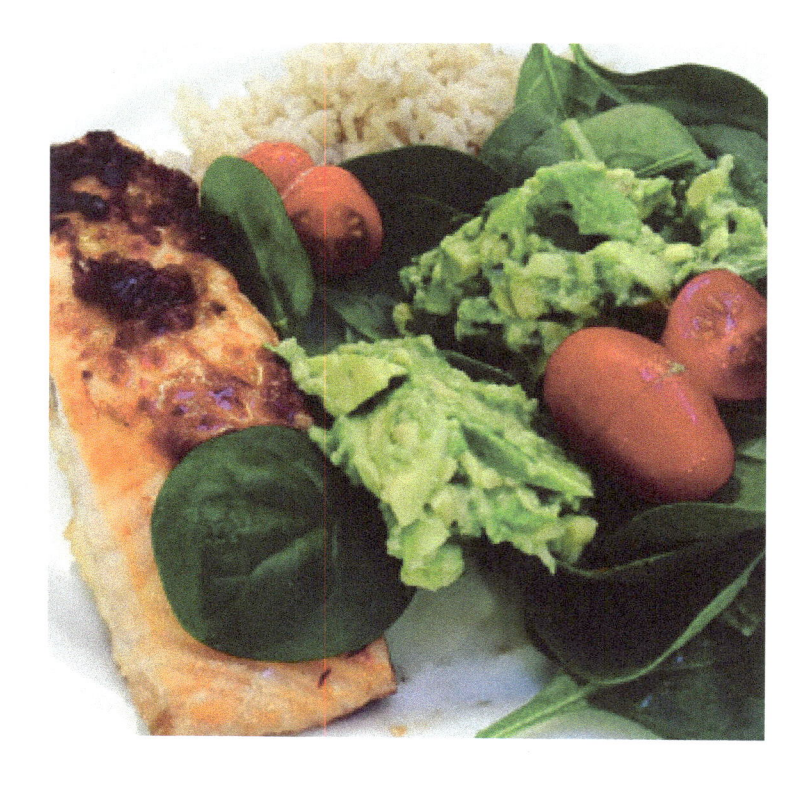

Baked scallops

This works well as a starter or a light lunch served with a salad and some Nutty Seed Bread.

Serves 4

1 large garlic clove, finely chopped
2 tbsp lemon juice
1 small bunch of flat leaf parsley, finely chopped
2 tbsp olive oil
12 scallops, coral on or off as you prefer
2-3 tsp butter

Preheat the oven to 220°C.

Mix the garlic, lemon juice, parsley and olive oil together and drizzle over the scallops. Season with sea salt and black pepper and blob a little butter on each.

Put the scallops on a baking tray (lined with baking parchment) and roast for 10 mins. or until tender.

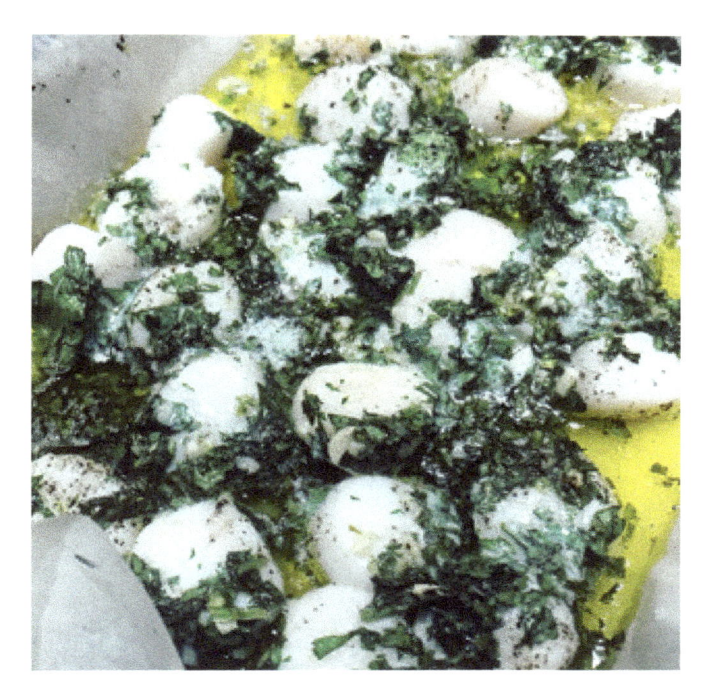

Meaty Mains

Chicken satay with vegetable noodles

This is my new signature dish, I have made it for so many friends and am always passing on the recipe. The satay sauce is worth making in its own right to go with vegetables anytime and keeps in the fridge for a good few days. This is easy despite the huge number of ingredients – I promise you will love it!

Serves 4

4 chicken breasts, cut into smaller fillets
2 tbsp curry powder
half Asian radish
1 large courgette
1 large carrot
1 large bunch of mint, leaves chopped
1 bunch of coriander, leaves chopped
1 bunch of Thai basil, leaves chopped

veggie dressing:
2 seeded red chillies
2-3 limes, juiced
2 tbsp fish sauce
1 tbsp coconut palm sugar

satay sauce:
1 tbsp olive oil
2 heaped tbsp Thai red curry paste
200ml coconut milk
200ml stock (I use Marigold bouillon)
4 tbsp unsweetened crunchy peanut butter (Whole Earth)
2 tbsp coconut palm sugar
1 tbsp fish sauce
1 tsp tamarind paste
4 lime leaves
juice of 1 lime

In a large bowl add the curry powder and a pinch of salt to the chicken pieces and mix until the chicken is coated all over. Leave to marinate while you prepare the noodles, veggie dressing and satay sauce. Spirilize the Asian radish, carrot and courgette into noodles.

Make the dressing by blending all the ingredients in a food processor. Pour the dressing over the vegetables.

Make the satay sauce by first heating the oil in a pan, add the curry paste and fry for a couple of minutes. Pour in the coconut milk and stock then add the peanut butter, sugar, fish sauce, tamarind paste, lime leaves and lime juice. Bring to the boil and then reduce heat and simmer for 5 mins. until you have a rich sauce.

Heat a griddle and grill the chicken for a few mins on each side until cooked through. Add the herbs to the noodles, toss together and place on a serving dish. When ready to serve reheat the sauce, place the chicken pieces on top of the noodles and drizzle the satay sauce over the dish.

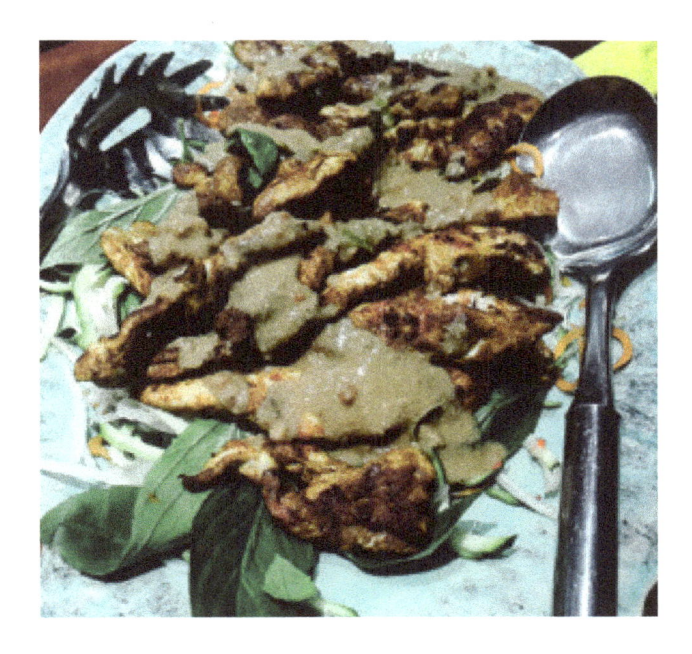

Turkey koftas with tahini dressing

Serves 4

3 spring onions, roughly chopped
2 green chillies, deseeded & finely chopped
3 garlic cloves, finely chopped
2 tsp ground coriander
2 tsp ground cumin
a pinch ground cloves
650g turkey mince
50g toasted pine nuts
1 large bunch of coriander, finely chopped
1 large bunch of parsley, finely chopped
1 tbsp olive oil

dressing:
2 tbsp tahini
6-8 tbsp boiling water
half a small garlic, finely chopped
150g natural yoghurt
3 tbsp freshly squeezed lemon juice
3 tbsp olive oil
half tsp sea salt
quarter tsp black pepper

This makes twice as much as you will need – but good to have in fridge – try over steamed vegetables or chunky white fish.

Place the spring onions, chillies, garlic, ground cumin, coriander and cloves in a blender, season with sea salt and black pepper and pulse to a paste. Place the turkey mince in a large bowl with the paste, pine nuts and fresh herbs. Mix well.

Shape the mix into approx. 16 small koftas and drizzle with the olive oil. Heat a grill/griddle, cook the koftas in batches, turning until browned on all sides. Cut one in half to check that is cooked through. If making in advance you can heat in a hot oven before serving.

To make the dressing, whisk the tahini and water together to form a smooth paste. Whisk in the rest of the ingredients.

Serve the koftas drizzled with the dressing and a big salad.

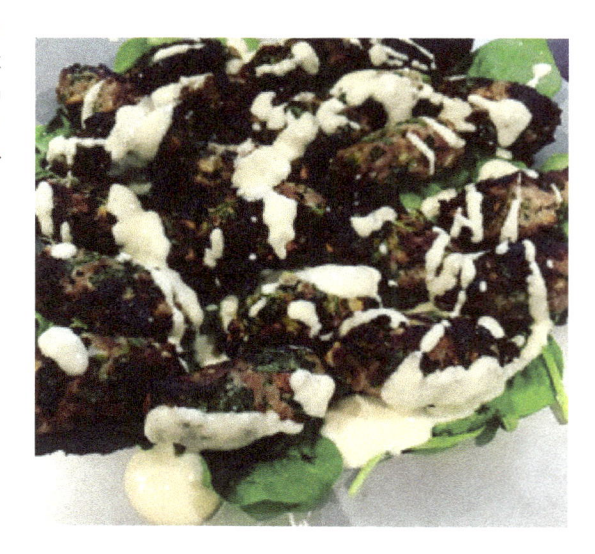

Marinated turkey breast

Serves 6

1 kg turkey breast - rolled

marinade:
4 tbsp parsley
4 tbsp coriander
4 tbsp mint leaves
1 garlic clove, peeled

4 tbsp lemon juice
4 tbsp olive oil
125ml white wine
half tsp ground cumin
half tsp sea salt
half tsp black pepper

Blend all the marinade ingredients in a food processor for a couple of minutes until smooth.

In a large bowl massage the marinde into the turkey breast, ensure that the meat is immersed in the marinade and cover the bowl. Leave in the fridge for 24 hours if possible.

Preheat the oven to 200°C and having removed the turkey from the marinade (saving this for later) roast in a roasting tray for 30 mins. Turn the oven down to 180°C and continue to roast until cooked through, (approx. 45 mins.) if necessary protecting the turkey with foil towards the end.

Heat the marinade for approx. 15 mins until reduced by half, seasoning to taste with salt and pepper. Serve the turkey thinly sliced covered with the sauce.

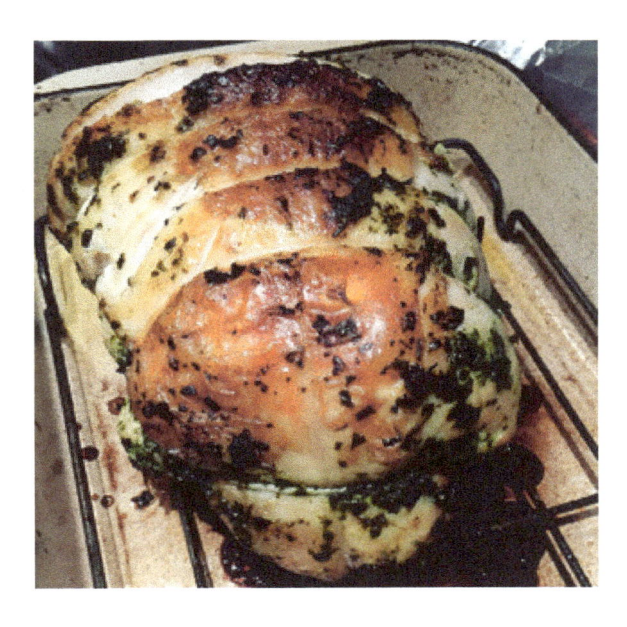

My favourite chicken curry

I tried this out using the same method as I use for Tarka Dahl and it works really well!

Serves 4-6

3 tbsp olive oil
1 tbsp cumin seeds
1 small onion, peeled & chopped
3-4 green chillies, slit with seeds removed
20g fresh ginger, peeled and cut into thin strips
4 chicken breasts, cut into bite size pieces

2 large cloves garlic, peeled
3-4 large tomatoes
sea salt
1 tsp turmeric
1 tsp garam masala
1 and half tsp ground coriander
handful fresh coriander leaves & stalks, chopped

Heat the oil in a large heavy based pan, add the cumin seeds and heat for a moment until fragrant. Add the onion, chillies and ginger and cook for about 10 mins until golden. Add the chicken pieces and stir well to brown the meat, this takes another 5 minutes.

Purée the garlic and tomatoes in a blender, add to the saucepan with the salt, powdered spices and a little water. Cook for about 15 mins. over a moderate heat, adding more water if necessary. If you like a thicker more creamy curry you could add a can of coconut milk and heat through.

Stir through the coriander and serve.

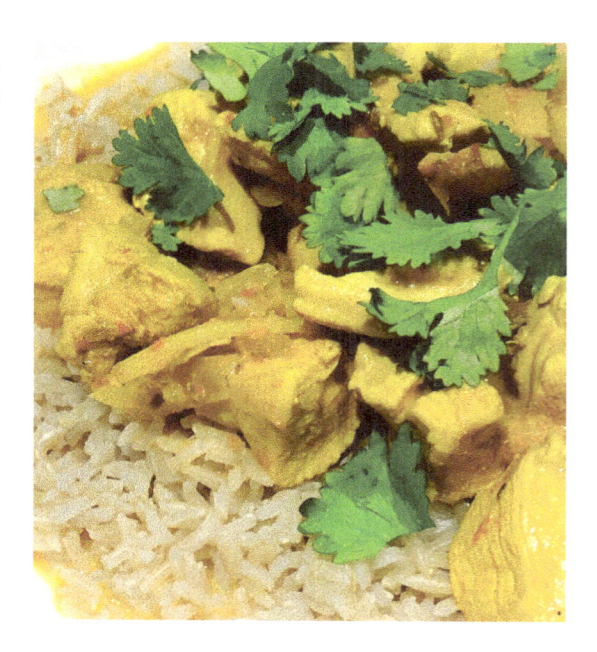

Grilled lamb with a herby salsa verde

Serves 4

1 tsp chilli flakes
1 tsp thyme leaves
half tsp ground cumin
sea salt & black pepper
2 tbsp olive oil
8 lamb cutlets (grass fed, organic)

salsa verde:
4 tbsp parsley
4 tbsp coriander
4 tbsp mint leaves
1 garlic clove, peeled
4 tbsp lemon juice
4 tbsp olive oil
125ml white wine
half tsp ground cumin
half tsp sea salt
half tsp black pepper
75ml extra virgin olive oil (5 tbsp)

Mix the chilli flakes, thyme, cumin, black pepper and a pinch of sea salt with the olive oil and pour this over the lamb. Leave to marinate while you make the salsa.

Place all the salsa ingredients into the food processor apart from the olive oil and pulse whilst slowly pouring in the olive oil.
Heat a griddle pan over a medium heat and cook the cutlets for about 4 mins on each side. Serve drizzled with the salsa verde and accompanied by a large green salad, green beans and some new potatoes.

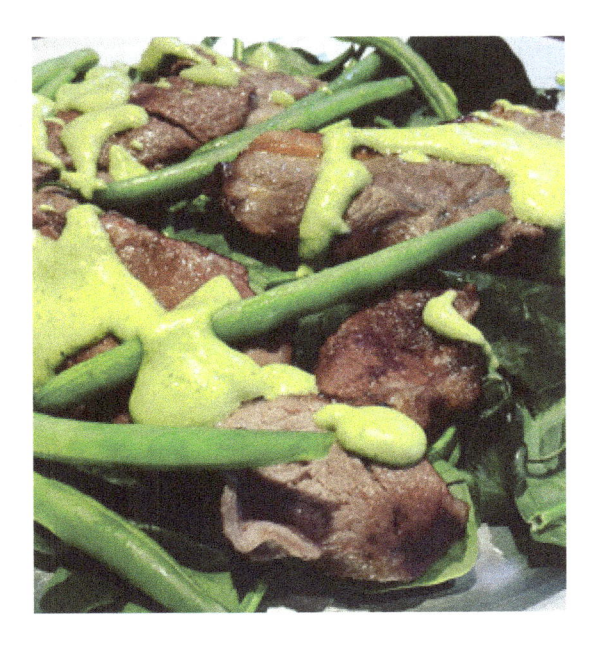

Chicken chimichurri

I like to make the chimichurri marinade the day before I need it - leaving it in the fridge overnight for the flavours to develop. Coat the chicken pieces in the marinade in the morning and then cook the dish in the evening for ultimate marination. If time is of the essence ignore all that and just marinate for as long as you can before cooking, it will still be delicious. The chimichurri also works really well with white fish.

Serves 4-6

4 organic chicken breasts cut into smaller fillets

chimichurri marinade:
1 jar or chargrilled peppers in oil, 350g drained (or the flesh of 3 roasted red peppers: roast peppers in the oven until charred, remove skin, deseed and slice)
1 small bunch of chives
1 small bunch of parsley
2 garlic cloves
pinch of oregano
sea salt & freshly ground black pepper
90 ml olive oil (6 tbsp)
2 tbsp white wine vinegar

Blitz the chimichurri ingredients in a food processor, transfer to a bowl, cover and leave in the fridge for the flavours to develop.

Put the chicken fillets into a shallow oven dish and pour over the chimichurri, using your hands or a spoon to make sure that all the chicken pieces are covered in the marinade.
Cover the dish and leave in the fridge to marinate until ready to cook. Preheat the oven to 180°C and cook the chicken for about 30 minutes (depending on size of fillets) so that it is cooked through.

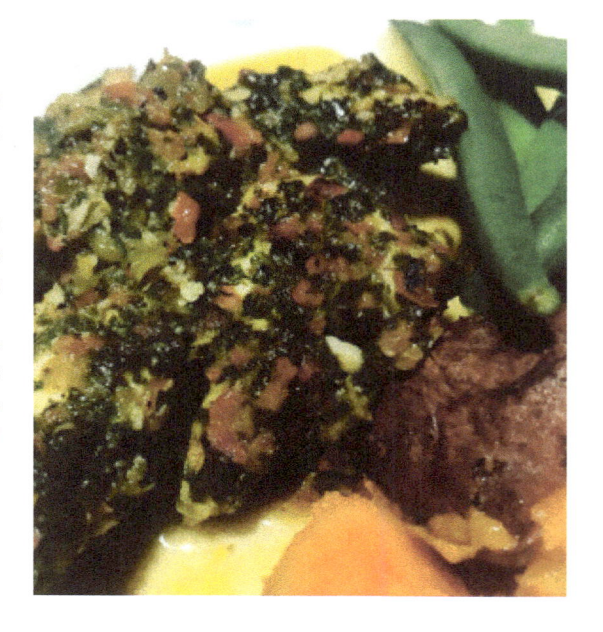

Minute steak with chicory & rocket salad and mayo dressing

Serves 4

1 head of chicory
1 shallot, thinly sliced
70g rocket
250g sirloin steak
extra virgin olive oil
20ml red wine vinegar

dressing:
1 egg yolk
2 tsp Dijon mustard
1 tbsp red wine vinegar
half garlic clove, finely chopped
100ml olive oil (7 tbsp)
2 tsp lemon juice
sea salt & black pepper

Cut the chicory in half lengthways and remove the core. Shred by slicing at an angle and combine with the shallot and rocket on a large platter.

Place the egg yolk, mustard, vinegar and garlic into a food processor. Add a pinch of sea salt and some black pepper. Blitz and whilst the blender is still running, slowly drizzle in the olive oil and then 2 tsp water and the lemon juice.

Slice the steak into thin ribbons, season with salt and black pepper and toss with a little olive oil. Heat a griddle pan until hot and cook the steak for a minute on each side (or longer if you prefer your meat more well done). Add the vinegar at the last minute and then set the steak aside. Dress the salad with 6 tbsp of the dressing. Serve the salad with the warm griddled steak on top.

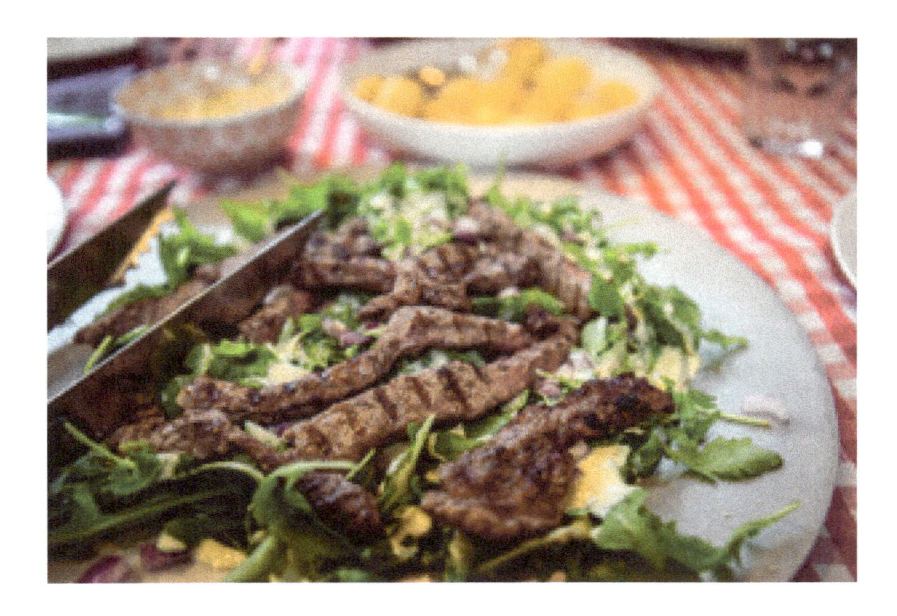

Two ways to roast chicken:

Roast chicken with butternut squash and sweet potato wedges

Serves 4

4 sweet potatoes
half a butternut squash
2 tbsp wholegrain mustard
2 lemons, juiced (keep the halves)
1 tbsp thyme leaves
4 tbsp olive oil

1 organic chicken (approx. 1.5kg)
2 red onions, peeled and cut into wedges
2 bay leaves
6 garlic cloves
125ml white wine

Preheat the oven to 180°C.

Combine the mustard, lemon juice, thyme and olive oil to make a marinade.

Halve the sweet potatoes lengthways and then cut each half into 4 giant chips. Cut the butternut squash into 1cm thick rings and halve these. Put the chicken, potatoes and squash, onion, bay leaves and 4 garlic cloves into a large oven dish. Season everything (including chicken cavity) with sea salt and black pepper. Put 2 of the squeezed lemon halves and the other 2 garlic cloves into the chicken cavity. Spread the marinade over the chicken and vegetables so that they are well covered. Pour a cup of water into the dish. Roast for 1 hour.

Pour the wine over the chicken, turn the vegetables and roast for another half hour, then turn the chicken onto it's breast for another 20 mins.

Check that the chicken is cooked throughly by pulling a leg away from the breast and making sure that the juices run clear and not bloody. Remove the chicken and vegetables to a warm dish, adding a little water if necessary to the oven dish to ensure there is a tasty 'gravy' to serve with the chicken. Serve hot or at room temperature with a big green salad.

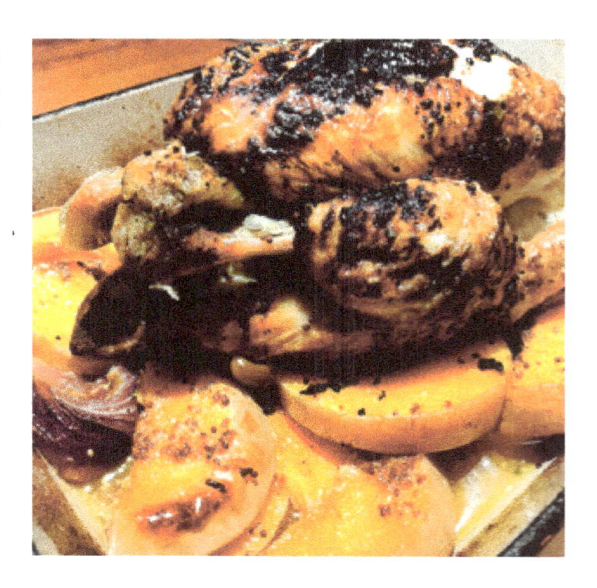

Harissa whole roast chicken

A simple and delicious way to prepare chicken – I love to do a couple of these when I have a large number of guests coming over - served along with jacket potatoes, humous, olives, taboulleh and a large mixed salad - my kind of food, so easy and everyone loves it.

1 organic whole chicken
1-2 tbsp harissa (Beluza rose harissa)
1 lemon

Pre heat the oven to 180°C.

Place your chicken on a rack in a roasting dish and rub the harissa into the skin so that the whole chicken is coated – you may prefer to wear disposable gloves for this (quite handy to keep in your kitchen for the really messy cooking jobs). Squeeze the juice of a lemon over the chicken and then put the lemon skins inside the chicken carcass. Place in the centre of the oven for about 1 and a half hours – depending on the size of your chicken – if you pull the leg away from the body the juices should run clear when the chicken is cooked through.

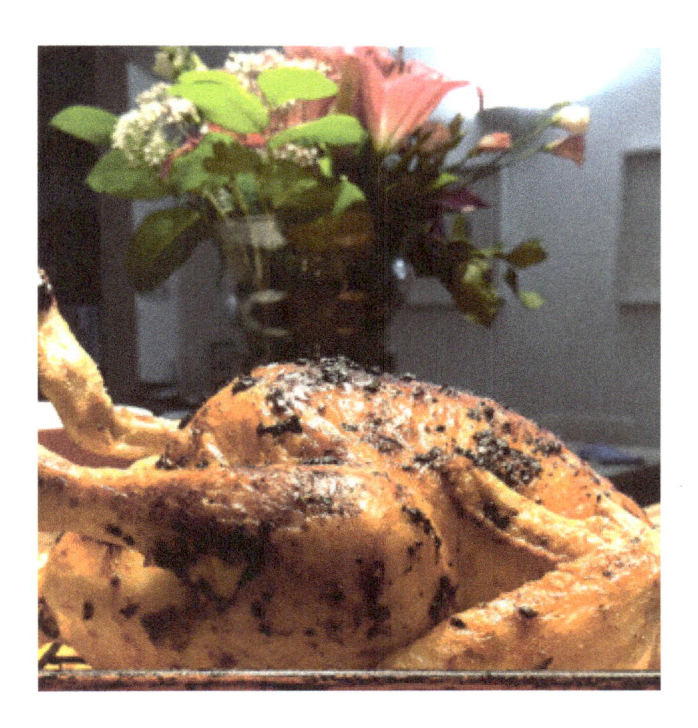

Veggie mains

Tofu Pad Prik

Serves 4

1 tbsp olive oil
250g firm tofu, cut into small squares (2cm)
2 tbsp Thai red curry paste
200g green beans, trimmed
1 red pepper, cut into strips
1 green pepper, cut into strips
75ml vegetables stock (Marigold)
half tbsp fish sauce
half tbsp fish sauce
half can coconut milk
half tsp coconut palm sugar
4 fresh kaffir lime leaves, finely sliced
large handful Thai basil leaves, torn
large handful of cashews, toasted in a dry pan

Heat the oil in a wok over a medium heat, add the tofu and sauté until golden on all sides. Set aside on kitchen paper. Add the curry paste to the wok and fry for 2 mins, then add the stock to thin the paste. Add the beans and peppers and sauté until tender. Add the coconut milk, fish sauce and sugar. Simmer for a few minutes and add back the tofu. Remove from the heat and add the kaffir leaves, Thai basil and cashew nuts. Serve with brown basmati rice.

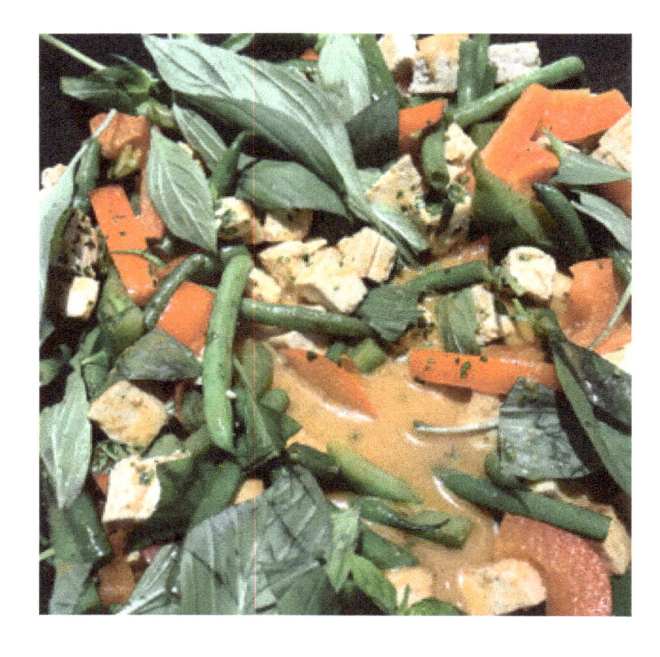

Beanotto with spinach

Beans are a good source of both protein and slow release carbs and therefore help to keep blood sugar levels stable – which helps with mood and energy balance. If you are OK with dairy a few tablespoons of mascarpone added at the end gives this dish added oomph.

Serves 4

extra virgin olive oil
1 large onion, finely chopped
2 garlic cloves, finely chopped
100g sliced mushrooms (oyster mushrooms work well)
120ml dry white wine
250g spinach, chopped
1 can cannellini beans
120ml stock (I use Marigold bouillon)
1 tbsp Engevita nutritional yeast flakes
grated zest and juice of half a lemon
handful of thyme leaves
sea salt & freshly ground black pepper

Sauté the onion and garlic in a little olive oil until softened. Add the mushrooms and stir in the wine and spinach and simmer until the spinach has wilted.

Add the beans and stock and continue to simmer for a few more minutes. Add the nutritional yeast flakes, lemon juice and thyme (and mascarpone if using). Season and serve sprinkled with a little lemon zest.

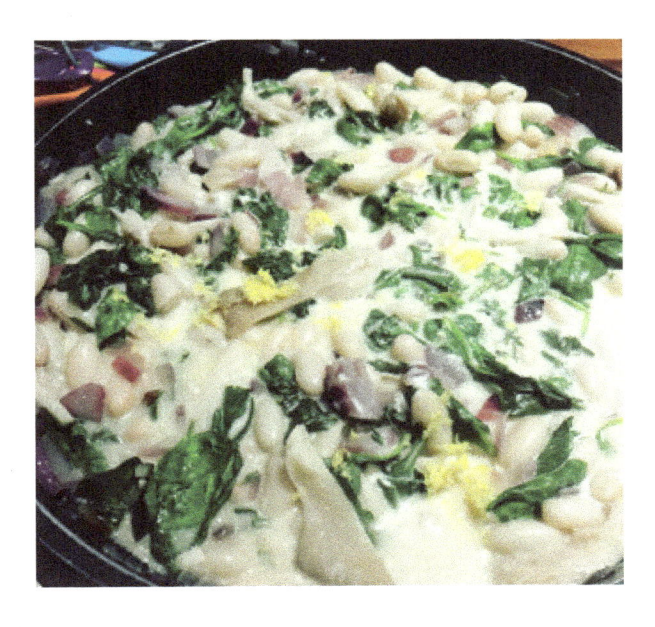

Quinoa burgers with tomato relish and tahini dressing

Serves 4

100g quinoa
(200g ready cooked quinoa)
200g frozen peas
1 x 400g can chickpeas
1 tsp ground cumin
1 tsp ground coriander
half tsp smoked paprika
4 dates
1 large bunch of fresh parsley
1 tbsp harissa
1 tsp Dijon mustard
50g sesame seeds

relish:
1 red onion, finely sliced
200g cherry tomatoes, chopped
balsamic vinegar
fresh coriander, chopped

dressing:
2 tbsp tahini
6-8 tbsp boiling water
half a small garlic, finely chopped
150g natural/ soya yoghurt
3 tbsp freshly squeezed lemon juice
3 tbsp olive oil
half tsp sea salt
quarter tsp black pepper

This makes twice as much as you will need – but good to have in fridge.

Preheat the oven to 180°C.

Toast the quinoa in a pan until it starts to pop and then add twice the volume of boiling water. Cook until all the water has been absorbed and the quinoa grains have released their curly 'tails'. Cover the peas with boiling water and allow to sit for 10 minutes.

Add the drained chickpeas to a frying pan with the ground cumin, coriander and paprika and toast until all the moisture has gone. Drain the peas and put in a dry bowl. Tip in half the chickpeas and half the cooked quinoa, add the dates, parsley, harissa and mustard and use a hand blender (or Magimix) to blitz the mixture until combined. Stir in the remaining chickpeas and quinoa and mix well. Form the mixture into 6 burgers and place on an oiled baking tray in the fridge whilst you make the relish.

Heat a little olive oil in a pan and fry the onion slowly for about 8 mins. Add the cherry tomatoes and cook for a further 5 mins. Add a dash of balsamic vinegar. Transfer to a bowl and add some coriander leaves.

Sprinkle the burgers with sesame seeds and bake in the oven for 20 mins.

To make the dressing whisk the tahini and water together to form a smooth paste. Whisk in rest of ingredients.

Serve the burgers on a bed of salad leaves with the tahini dressing and relish.

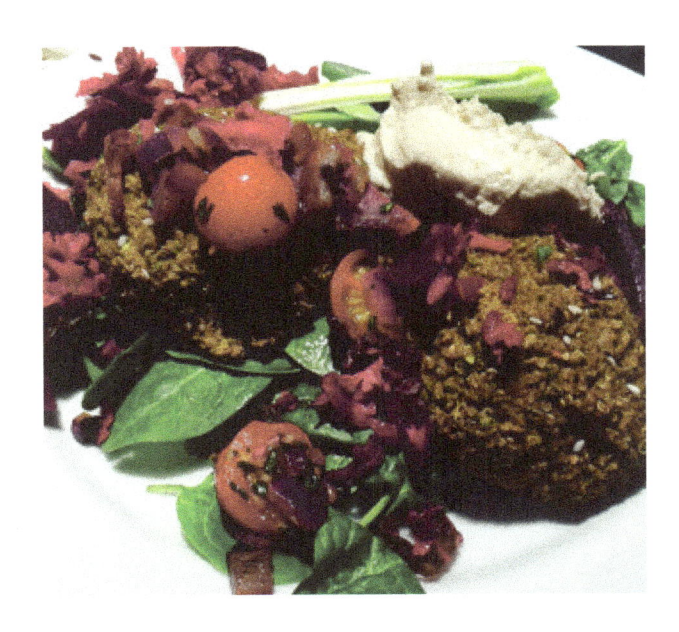

Chickpea and kale hotpot

Serves 4

1 x can chickpeas, drained
4 cloves garlic, peeled
1 thumb sized piece of fresh ginger, peeled
5 tbsp olive oil
1 onion, diced
4 bay leaves
1 tbsp coriander seeds, ground
half tsp dried chilli powder
4 sprigs rosemary
3 sprigs sage
2 cans tomatoes
1 butternut squash, peeled and chopped
400ml vegetables stock (Marigold)
120g kale, washed and chopped
handful frozen peas
half lemon

Smash the garlic and ginger to a paste in a pestle and mortar.

Heat the oil in a large pan, cook the onions very slowly with a good pinch of salt and the bay leaves for approx. 15 mins covered with a lid.

Stir through the garlic and ginger and then add the coriander, chilli, herbs, tomatoes and squash, cook covered for another 15 mins until the squash is tender. Stir in the chickpeas, add the stock and bring to the boil. Cook on a gentle heat for another 30 mins. Stir through the kale and peas until the kale has wilted and the peas have heated through.

Squeeze over the lemon juice and check seasoning before serving.

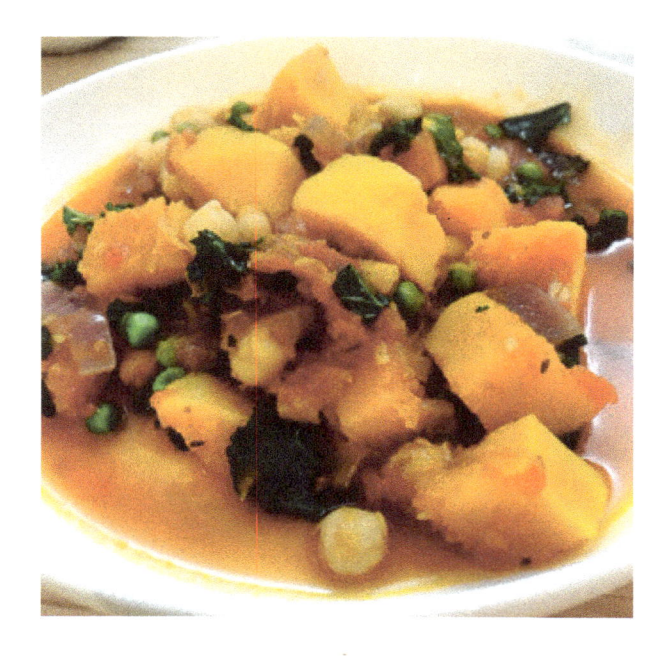

Veggie bolognaise

Make this in bulk and freeze as it is such a great recipe, the nutritional yeast gives a 'cheese' taste without cheese and provides important B vitamins which are good for boosting metabolism. In theory you could do all the chopping by hand but a food processor makes life much easier.

Serves 4

- 1 head of cauliflower
- 2 carrots, peeled
- 200g mushrooms
- 1 medium onion
- 3 cloves garlic
- 125g walnuts
- 2 x 400g cans chopped tomatoes
- 20g sundried tomatoes
- 2 tbsp Engevita nutritional yeast
- 1 tsp dried oregano
- sea salt & freshly ground black pepper

Soak the sundried tomatoes in a bowl by covering with warm water.

Use a food processor to grate the carrot and then pulse the cauliflower, mushrooms, onion and garlic to a fine texture. You may have to do this in a few batches, depending on the size of your food processor bowl. Heat a large pan and gently sauté the vegetables in 1 tbsp olive oil until they are soft and reduced in size, you can add a little water to the vegetables if they start to stick.

Grind the walnuts in the food processor to a coarse texture and add to the vegetables with the salt, oregano and nutritional yeast. Stir well.

Drain the sundried tomatoes and put in the food processor with 1 can of tomatoes, puree until smooth and then add to the vegetables in the pan with the second can of chopped tomatoes. Season with salt and pepper and add a teaspoon of coconut sugar or maple syrup if too acidic. Simmer for 15 minutes on a gentle heat, stirring occasionally. Serve with courgette spaghetti.

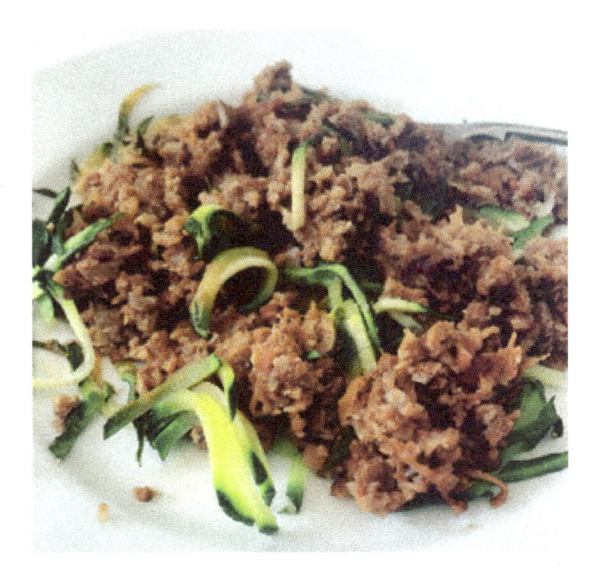

Coconut and chickpea curry

Serves 4

3 cardamom pods
3 onions, finely chopped
4 cloves of garlic, finely chopped
2cm piece of ginger, finely chopped
2 fresh green chillies, finely chopped
extra virgin olive oil
1/2 cinnamon stick
2 cloves
1 pinch of fennel seeds
1/2 tsp ground turmeric
1 level tsp chilli powder
1 heaped tsp ground coriander
1 level tsp garam masala
1 heaped tsp tomato purée
4 ripe tomatoes
2 x 400g cans chickpeas
1 bunch of fresh coriander
200ml coconut milk
100g baby spinach or kale

Place a heavy based, large pan over a medium heat to get hot. Crush the cardamom pods to release the seeds.

Pour a good drizzle of oil into the pan, add the cinnamon, cardamom, cloves and fennel seeds. Then add the garlic, ginger and green chillies.

Stir fry for a couple of minutes, then add the onion. Cook for a further 15 to 20 minutes, or until soft and golden, stirring occasionally.

Add the turmeric, chilli powder, ground coriander, garam masala, tomato purée and a pinch of sea salt and stir so that everything is well combined.

Chop and add the tomatoes, then pour in 400ml water (or less for a thicker curry). Bring to the boil. Drain and rinse the chickpeas and add to the pan.

With the lid on cook over a medium heat for 15 minutes, stirring occasionally.

Pick and finely chop the coriander leaves, and set aside to garnish.

Reduce the curry to a low heat and pour in the coconut milk. Simmer gently for 5 minutes, until well combined, adding the spinach/kale to wilt for the last couple of minutes.

Season with sea salt and black pepper. Remove the pan from the heat, scatter with the reserved coriander and serve with some brown basmati rice.

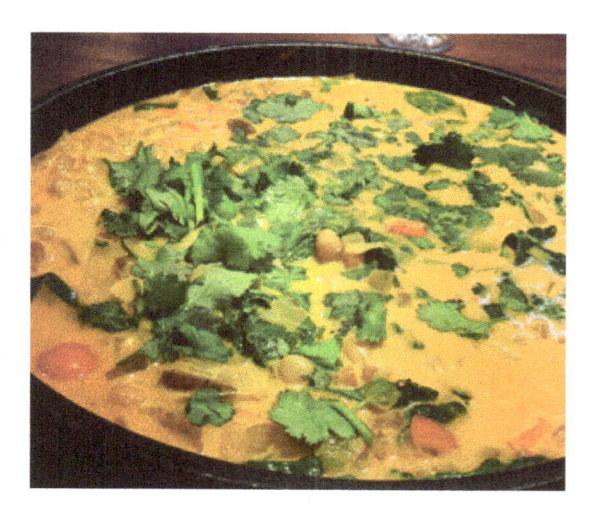

Cauliflower based pizza

This is an excellent way of incorporating the cruciferous vegetables cauliflower and rocket into your diet – these vegetables support liver detox.

Serves 2

1 cauliflower
2 eggs
sea salt
1 tbsp of oregano
3 tbsp of quinoa flour (or other wholegrain gluten free flour)
1 x 400g can tomatoes
1 tsp of dried rosemary
1 white onion
coconut oil
100g rocket
asparagus spears
olives, artichoke hearts

Preheat the oven to 180°C.

Remove the green stalks from the cauliflower, cut the cauliflower into smaller pieces and pulse in the food processor until it is finely minced.

In a bowl combine the chopped cauliflower with the eggs, a large pinch of salt, the oregano and gluten free flour. Mix together to form a dough and split into two. Place one half on baking paper and flatten out with a spoon or spatula until you form a circle just under 1cm in thickness. Repeat with other half.

Melt 2 tsp of coconut oil on a medium heat or use olive oil and brush the oil over the pizza bases. Place them both in the oven to cook for 20 mins.

Make the topping by cutting the white onion up very small, sauté it in 1 tbsp of coconut oil/olive oil with the rosemary on a medium heat with a pinch of sea salt for 5 minutes. Add in the can of tomatoes and cook for another 5-10 minutes.

Steam a handful of asparagus spears. By this time it will be time to take the bases out.

Spoon the tomato mix on top of the bases and cook for another 5 minutes until the edges crisp (but don't burn). Take them out and distribute the rocket, asparagus, olives and artichoke halves evenly over the pizzas.

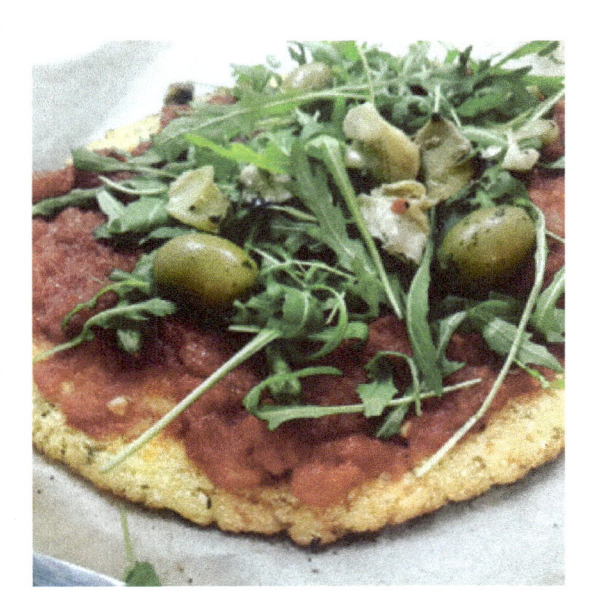

Gado Gado

This dish is well worth the effort – it is so delicious and full of vegetables so supplies plenty of antioxidants to enhance your health.

Serves 6

peanut sauce:
1 tbsp olive oil
2 heaped tbsp Thai curry paste
200ml coconut milk
200ml stock
4 tbsp crunchy peanut butter (Whole Earth unsweetened)
2 tbsp coconut sugar
1 tbsp fish sauce
1 tsp tamarind paste
4 kaffir lime leaves
1 lime, juiced

Gado Gado:
2 tbsp cold-pressed coconut oil
1/2 small head savoy cabbage, shredded
1/2 small head red cabbage, shredded
6-7 kale leaves, hard 'stalk' removed and leaves sliced into ribbons
2 medium sweet potato, in slim wedges
4 carrots, spiralized
200g bean shoots/spouts either shop-bought or home-grown (see vegan gut week for instructions)
2 shallots, sliced into rings
1 small bunch coriander, roughly chopped
a few pinches sea salt
limes for serving

Make the satay sauce by first heating the oil in a pan, add the curry paste and fry for a couple of minutes. Pour in the coconut milk and stock then add the peanut butter, sugar, fish sauce, tamarind paste, lime leaves and lime juice. Bring to the boil and then reduce heat and simmer for 5 mins. until you have a rich sauce.

Set a steamer over boiling water and place the sweet potato inside, cover, and steam for approx 6 minutes until tender. Remove from the steamer and toss with a little of the coconut oil, then cover to keep warm. Next place the carrots, kale and cabbage in the steamer and cook for 2-4 minutes until tender-crisp, then toss with remaining coconut oil. In a large bowl combine all the steamed vegetables with shoots/sprouts, shallots and coriander. Sprinkle with salt and toss together. Arrange the Gado Gado vegetables on a plate and add a generous serving of the peanut sauce, serve with a wedge of lime. You may like to top with some tempeh.

Peanut sauce keeps in the fridge for a few days and is delicious on everything!

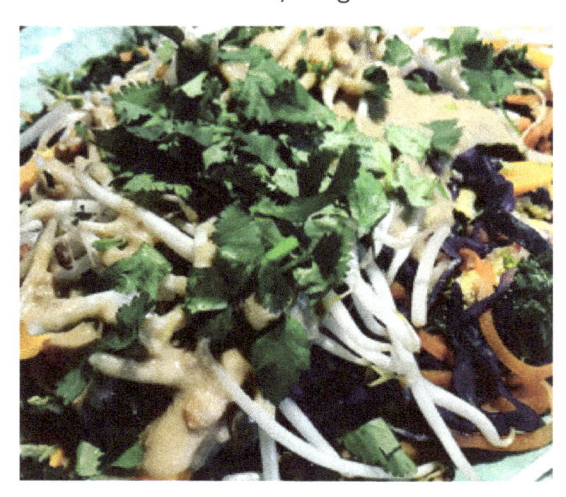

Sweet Things

I love a cup of tea with a piece of one of these cakes or one of these special desserts after dinner. I don't ban all sugar from my house as I really believe that it is all about balance and knowing when to stop – ideally after one serving! Once you are eating healthily and are in good health you can allow yourself a treat now and then especially if it is made with good wholesome ingredients as in the recipes below – just don't overdo it!

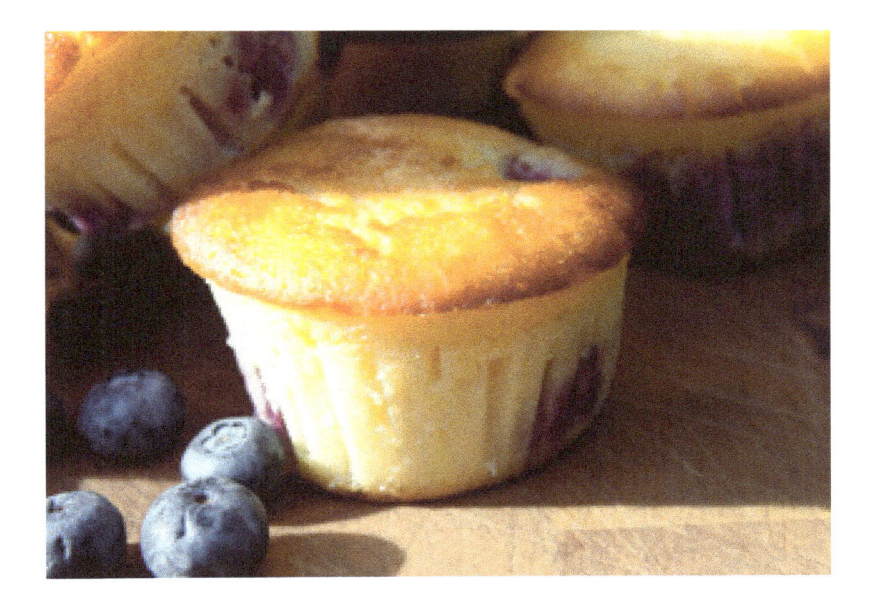

Chocolate avocado mousse

This is a bit Marmite – you either love it or hate it, I have experimented a lot and I think this version of the recipe works brilliantly.

Serves 2-4

1 large ripe avocado
3 tbsp raw cacao powder
4 dates, pitted
1 large ripe banana, peeled (and frozen if you want to eat immediately)
half tsp of good quality vanilla extract
2 tbsp water

Place all the ingredients into a high-speed blender and blend until you have a smooth mixture. Divide into ramekin dishes or pretty tea cups and decorate with a mint leaf or a few berries.

These keep well in the fridge if you are making for later.

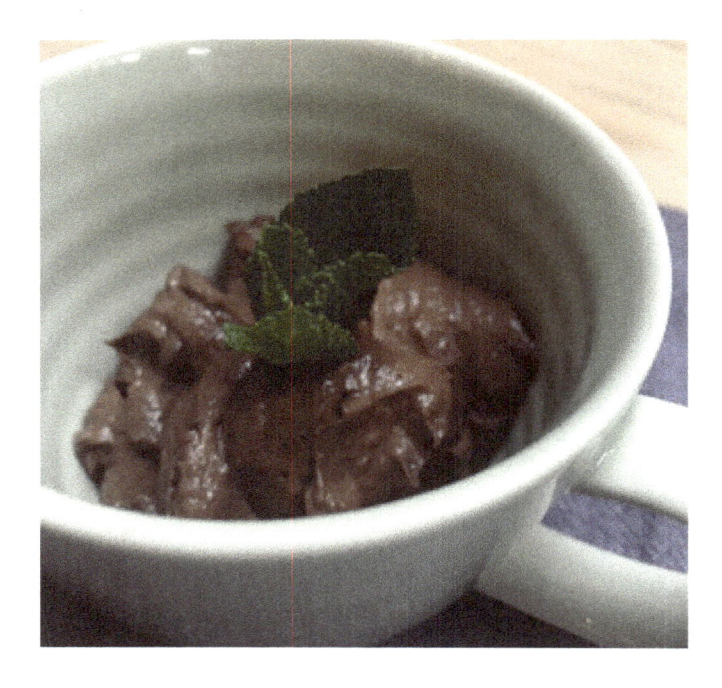

Nutty chocolate ice cream

This is so good I wish I could package it and sell it but it needs to be eaten immediately. I have given this to guests at dinner parties and they really love it – they can't believe it's actually quite nutritious!

Whenever you have bananas that are going over to the dark side you should peel, slice and freeze them as it's great to have frozen bananas at the ready for this recipe as well as for the mousse above and for smoothies. If you don't fancy this banana version the recipe works well with frozen mango or pineapple.

Serves 2

3 bananas, peeled, sliced and pre frozen
1 tbsp raw cacoa
1 tbsp maple syrup
2 tbsp almond milk
1 tbsp almond butter
half tsp vanilla extract

Put everything into a powerful blender (Vitamix for example) and blitz until smooth.

Serve immediately with some chopped pecans/almonds and some cacoa nibs.

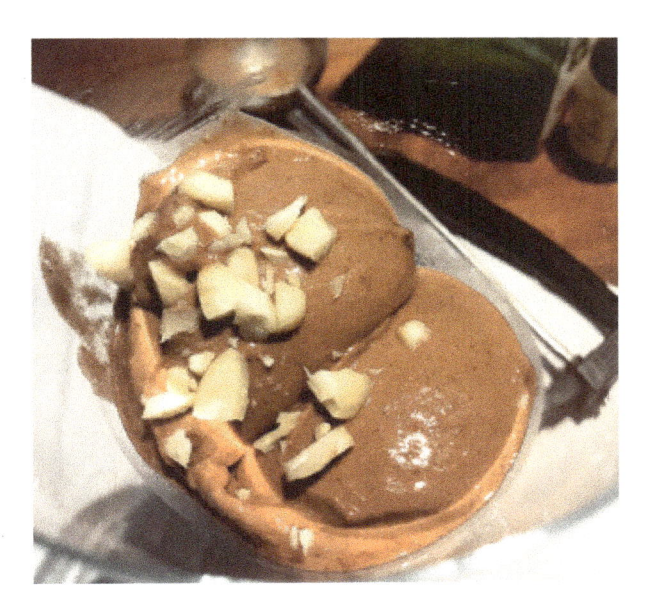

Energy balls

There are lots of versions of this recipe online and in all the current healthy cook books but I don't think you need to overcomplicate things; no need to add honey as the dried fruit is sweet enough and no need to add coconut oil as the mixture binds perfectly well if you blend the nuts for long enough or soak them overnight. If you are an all or nothing person you should probably freeze the balls and just take out a couple a day – they are quite moreish. Perfect for a lunch box snack or an after dinner treat.

They also make great presents to take along to dinner with friends.

10 small pitted dates
10 figs, hard stalk removed
50g good quality cocoa/raw cacoa
25g ground almonds or ground flaxseeds
200g cashew nuts
25g hemp protein powder – optional

Put the cashews in a bowl and cover with water, leave to soak for at least 2 hours or overnight. Drain and rinse with fresh water. Blitz in a food processor to a fine crumb texture.

Put the rest of the ingredients in the food processor and continue to blend until the mixture holds together and has a chunky, sticky consistency. (If the mixture is too dry you can add a little almond butter so that it comes together).

Roll the mixture into small balls – and then roll in cacoa so that they look just like chocolate truffles. Alternatively you can press into a lined baking tray, cut into squares and refrigerate ready for lunchboxes/treats.

For variety you can use different nuts and dried fruits, you can also add different superfoods: maca, spirulina, bee pollen... vary what you use every time and you will never get bored of these little balls of loveliness.

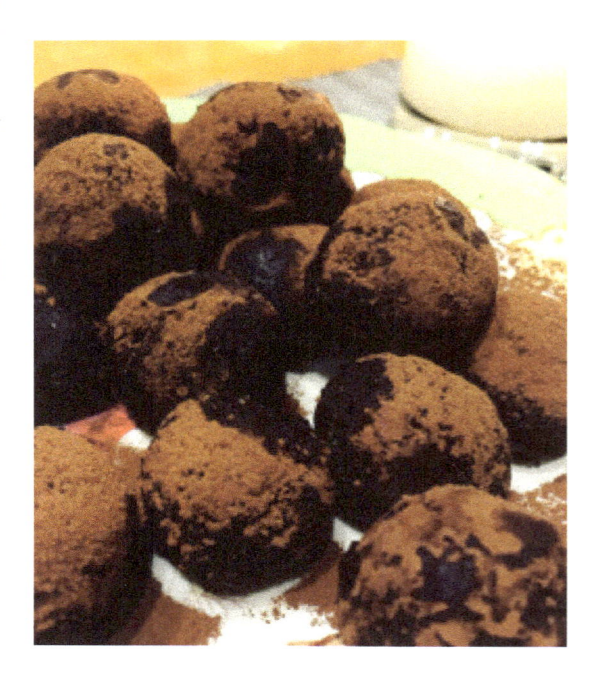

Hazelnut and blueberry mini muffins

These are the perfect size to put on your saucer with a cup of tea – just enough of a treat.

Makes 24 bite sized muffins

100g unsalted butter (melted & cooled)
25g Infinity foods brown rice flour
or Infinity Foods corn flour
45g ground almonds
45g ground hazelnuts
1 vanilla pod, slit and seeds removed
(or 1 tsp vanilla extract)

3 large egg whites
125g maple syrup
zest of an unwaxed lemon
85g blueberries

Preheat oven to 180°C. Grease the muffin tray with a little butter.

Mix the flour, ground nuts and vanilla seeds in a bowl.

In a separate clean bowl whisk the egg whites to a light floppy foam.

Make a well in the middle of the dry ingredients and tip in the egg whites, the melted butter and syrup. Add the zest and stir to a light batter.

Spoon the mixture into the muffin tray and place a blueberry on top of each muffin. Bake for 15 mins. Cool for 5 mins. and then turn onto a wire rack.

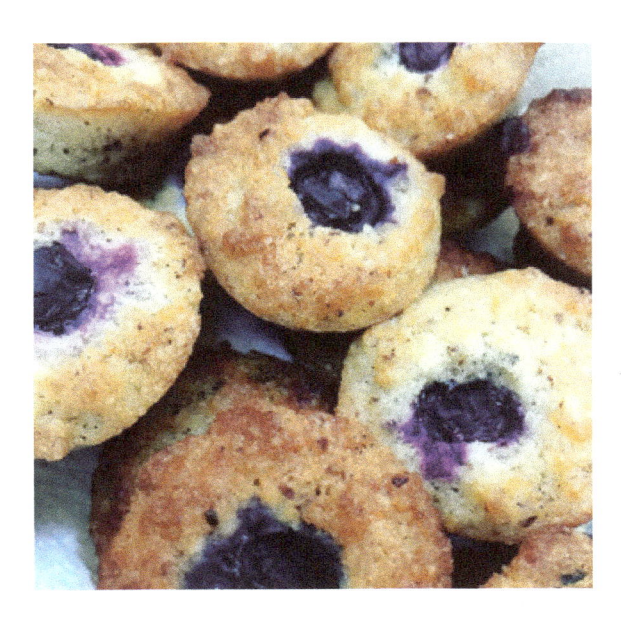

Light and easy Christmas pudding

I have been making this same pudding for years, it is so delicious and not as heavy as traditional pudding as it doesn't contain suet. You make it in a pudding bowl but bake it in the oven like a cake. In fact why wait until Christmas?

Serves 8

275g raisins
175g chopped dates
100g chopped figs
100g sultanas
9 tbsp orange juice
100g gluten free breadcrumbs
225g butter
175g coconut palm sugar

grated rind of 1 lemon and 1 orange
4 beaten eggs
50g chopped almonds
100g brown rice flour
2 tsp baking powder
1 tsp mixed spice
1 tsp cinnamon

Grease a 1.5 litre pudding basin. Line the base with a circle of greaseproof paper. Pre heat oven to 180°C.

Place the dried fruits and 5 tbsp of orange juice in a pan, cover and simmer for 5 mins. Place in a large bowl and add the breadcrumbs.

Beat the butter and sugar together until creamy, then beat in the lemon and orange rind, eggs, almonds, flour and spices. Add this to the fruit mixture and mix until everything is well combined. Pack the mixture into the pudding basin and cover with greaseproof paper. Bake for 1 hour and 20 mins. until springy yet firm to touch – test the centre is cooked by putting a skewer into the middle of the pudding – it should come out clean – if not then replace in the oven for a little longer and keep checking, you may need to cover the top with foil to prevent it from burning.

Pour over the remaining orange juice. Turn out and serve decorated with shredded lemon and orange zest.

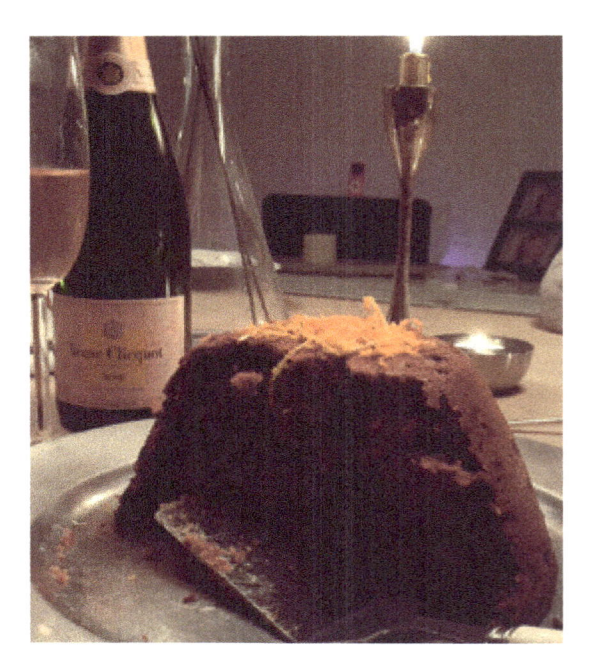

Chocolate red velvet cake

The dark red colour comes from beetroot which is great for liver health and a good source of iron. This is my all time favourite cake, great as a dinner party pudding but also amazing with an afternoon cup of tea.

200g cooked, unseasoned beetroot, peeled and puréed
4 large eggs
4 tbsp maple syrup
1 tsp vanilla extract
1 tbsp raw cacoa powder
1 tsp baking powder
pinch salt
125g ground almonds
125g dark chocolate – 70% cocoa
4 tbsp olive oil

Preheat oven to 180°C and line a 22cm loose bottomed cake tin.

In a large mixing bowl, beat the beetroot, eggs, maple syrup, vanilla extract, cocoa powder, baking powder and salt. Fold in the ground almonds.

Place a bowl on top of a saucepan of simmering water and melt the chocolate, mix in the oil. Gently stir this mixture into the cake mixture.

Scrape the mixture into the tin and bake for 35-40 mins. until a skewer comes out clean. Leave the cake to cool in the tin before turning out onto a wire rack. Once cooled dust the cake with a little cocoa powder and decorate with berries. Serve with crème fraîche or natural/coconut milk yoghurt.

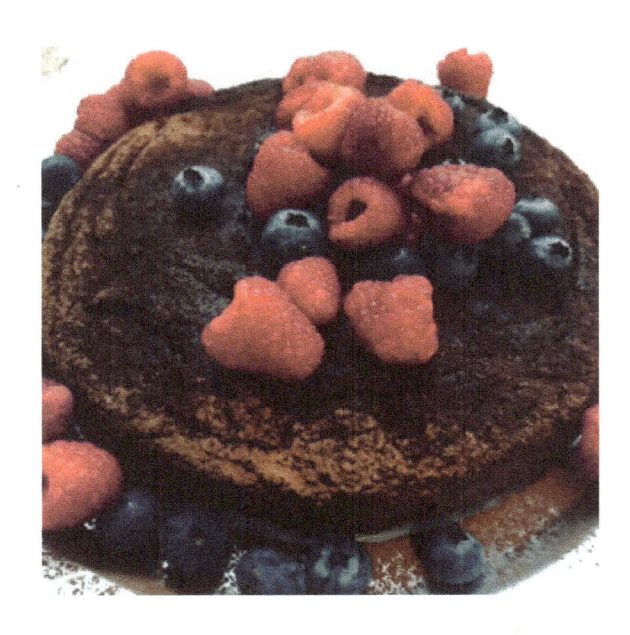

Flapjack muffins

My husband and 2 boys absolutely love these flapjack muffins – they started calling them 'Man Buns' as a joke and as they like to think they are a more manly muffin, my Mum now calls them this which makes us all giggle! Great for car journeys or if you have missed breakfast – be warned they are very filling!

Makes 12 generous muffins

300g gluten free oats
225g gluten free flour
half tsp baking powder
2 tsp sea salt
50g ground flax seeds
85g chopped walnuts
70g coconut oil

85g unsalted butter
150ml maple syrup
2 large eggs, lightly beaten
1 tsp ground cinnamon
1 tsp vanilla extract
handful raisins

Preheat the oven to 160°C.

Butter a standard 12 cup muffin tin.

Combine the oats, flour, baking powder, salt, flax seeds, cinnamon, raisins and walnuts in a large bowl.

In a medium saucepan, over a low heat combine the coconut oil, butter, vanilla extract and syrup and slowly melt together.

Pour the melted mixture over the oat mixture. Stir, add the eggs and combine to a wet dough. Spoon the dough into the muffin tin, I use an ice-cream scoop – to three quarters full.

Bake for 25 mins. in the top third of the oven until golden. Remove from the oven and allow to cool for 5 mins in the tin. Tip out onto a rack to completely cool.

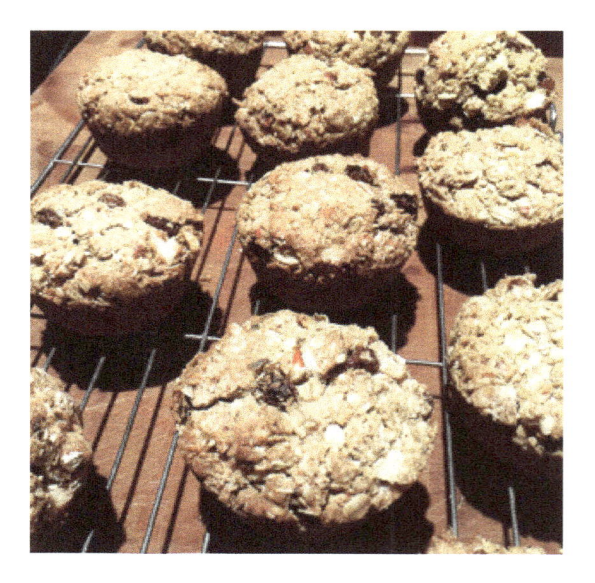

Lemon berry muffins

These muffins featured in my first book and were so popular that I thought they should appear again. They are very light and utterly delicious with an afternoon cup of tea.

60g butter
100g Infinity Foods corn flour
(from health food shop –
not the white thickening agent)
100g ground almonds
2 rounded tsp baking powder
150g coconut palm sugar
juice and zest of 1 unwaxed lemon
120ml milk – almond /cow's – your choice
1 large egg
150g fresh or frozen raspberries/blueberries

Preheat oven to 200°C.

Melt the butter in a small saucepan and leave to cool.

Stir together the corn flour, almonds, baking powder, sugar and lemon zest.

In a measuring jug combine the lemon juice and enough milk to reach the 200ml mark, then beat in the egg and melted butter.

Pour the milk mixture into the dry ingredients and stir together briefly. Fold in the berries and spoon the mixture into a greased 12-bun muffin tray.

Bake for approx 25 minutes, leave to cool in the tray for 5 minutes and then turn out onto a rack and cool thoroughly.

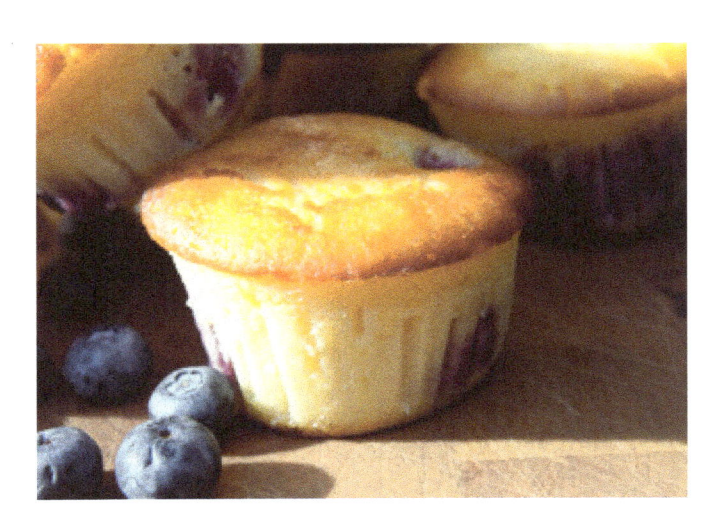

Raspberry cashew 'cheese' cake

I couldn't produce a cookery book in 2019 without a cashew 'cheese cake', these are very de rigueur and make an impressive dessert.

the crust:
100g raw almonds (or pecans/walnuts)
150g soft dates
quarter tsp sea salt

the filling:
200g raw cashews, soaked overnight and drained
juice of 1 lemon
the seeds of 1 vanilla bean
 (or 1tsp vanilla extract)
200g full fat Greek yoghurt
 (or coconut yoghurt)
3-4 tbsp maple syrup
200g raspberries/summer berries – fresh or frozen

Place nuts and dates in a food processor with sea salt and pulse to a fine texture. Test the crust by spooning out a small amount of mixture and rolling it in your hands. If the ingredients hold together, your crust is perfect, if it doesn't then add some almond butter. Spoon crust mixture into a 20cm spring-form tin, and press firmly, making sure that the edges are well packed and that the base is relatively even throughout. Put in the fridge to set.

Rinse food processor well. Place all filling ingredients (except the berries) in the food processor and blend on high until very smooth (this make take a couple minutes so be patient).

Pour about 2/3 of the mixture out onto the crust and smooth with a spatula. Add the berries to the remaining filling and blend on high until smooth. Pour onto the first layer of filling. Place in freezer until solid. To serve, remove from freezer 30 minutes prior to eating. Run a smooth, sharp knife under hot water and cut the cheesecake into slices. Serve on its own, or with fresh fruit. Store leftovers in the freezer.

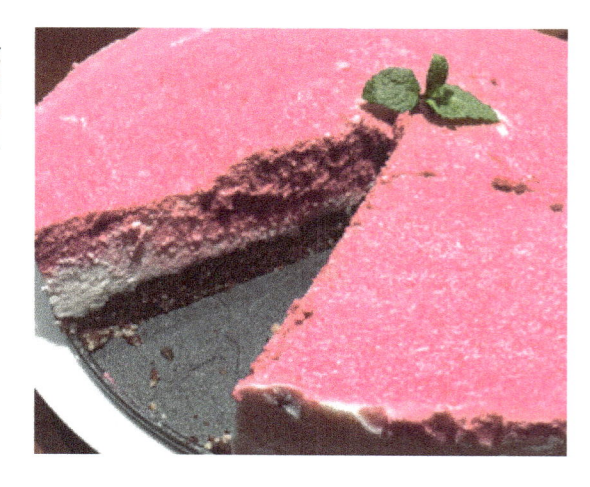

Poached nectarines with ginger cashew cream

Serves 6

8 nectarines, cut in half and stones removed
300ml pomegranate juice (carton)
2 star anise
2 cinnamon sticks

ginger cashew cream:
125g cashew nuts
2 tbsp coconut oil
juice of one large orange
2cm piece of fresh root ginger, peeled and grated

Put the nectarines, pomegranate juice, star anise and cinnamon sticks in a saucepan. Bring to the boil and then simmer for 5 mins or until the fruit is soft.

To make the cream, put all the ingredients into a blender and process until smooth, adding a little water to thin if necessary.

Serve the nectarines either hot or cold with the cream. This will keep in the fridge for up to 3 days.

The cream is great over any dessert – it would be good with the Christmas pud.

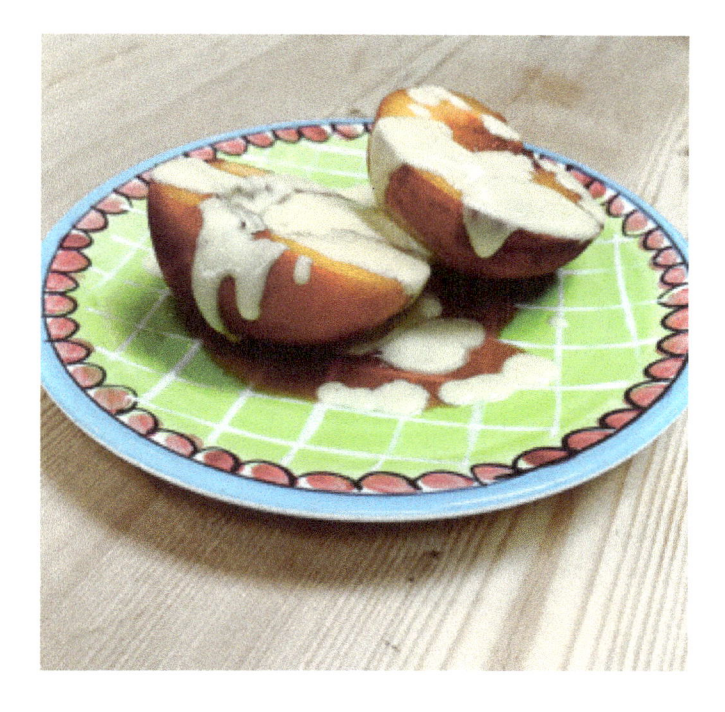

Baked apples

Baked apples make a great dessert but are also amazing for breakfast – hot or cold. Baked or stewed apples are really good for gut health as they help to heal the gut lining.

Serves 4

4 medium sized Bramley apples
2 tbsp ground almonds
2 tbsp organic raisins

1 tbsp chopped walnuts
1 tbsp butter
1 tbsp maple syrup

Core and make a slit around the circumference of each apple. Fill the centre of each apple with a mixture of ground almonds, chopped walnuts and raisins. Place the apples in a baking dish and drizzle a little maple syrup over the top of each apple and top with a blob of butter. Put a little water into the bottom of the dish and place in the oven for approx. 40 mins. Keep an eye on the apples as they go from perfect to sherbet in what seems like seconds. They are ready when a skewer goes through the flesh with ease.

Serve with natural/coconut milk yoghurt.

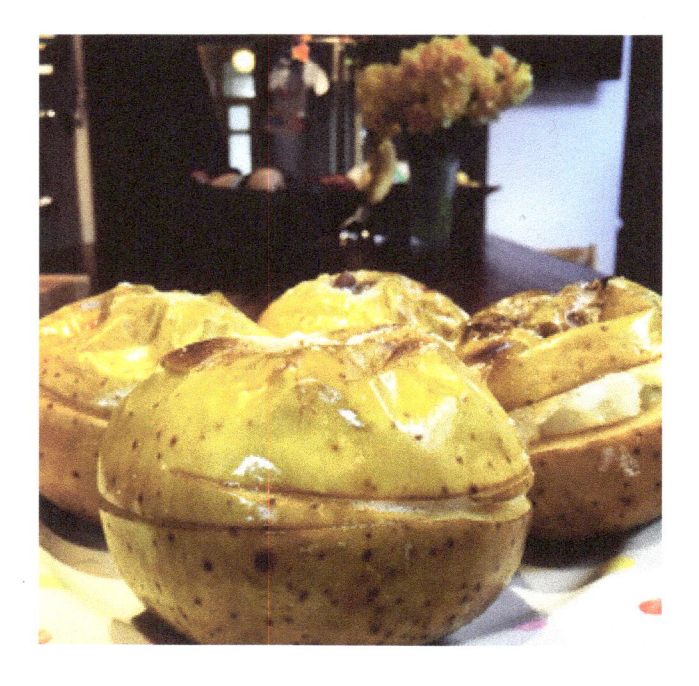

Mangoes and pineapple in chilli syrup

This is a wonderfully refreshing dessert, great after a hot curry or as a Summer pud.

Serves 4

2 large ripe mangoes
1 large ripe pineapple
4 tbsp maple syrup
zest and juice of 2 limes

1 star anise
1 red chilli, deseeded and finely chopped
torn mint leaves

Skin and dice the mangoes and pineapple and place in a bowl. Put the syrup, lime zest and juice, star anise and chilli into a small pan and bring to simmering point. Simmer gently for 5 minutes and then allow the liquid to cool.

When the syrup is cool, pour over the fruit and marinate in the fridge for about 45 mins. Sprinkle with torn mint leaves before serving.

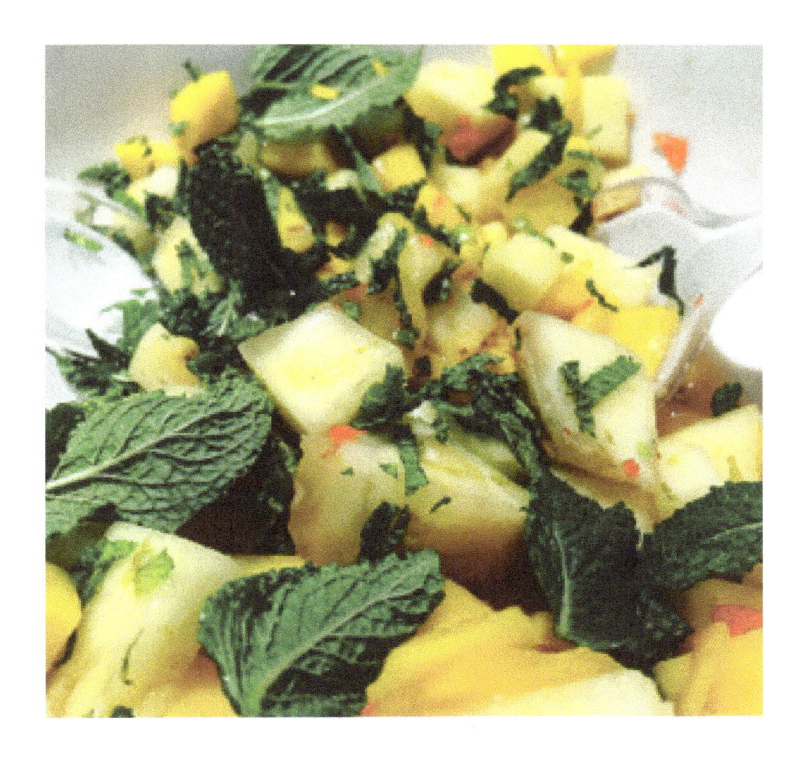

Poached pears with raw chocolate sauce

I love to make this, the chocolate sauce is magical and ridiculously easy to make. Quite an impressive dessert for minimum effort.

Serves 4

8 rooibos tea bags –
Earl Grey rooibos works well
3 tbsp pure maple syrup
4 firm, ripe pears, peeled and sliced lengthwise, cored

for the sauce:
3 tbsp olive oil
1 1/2 tbsp pure maple syrup
pinch fine sea salt
3 tbsp raw cacoa

Bring a litre of water to boil in a medium saucepan and add the tea, remove from heat and steep for 15 mins. Remove the teabags and sweeten the tea with the maple syrup.

Return the pan to the heat and bring to a simmer. Add the pears and simmer for 20 mins.

Whisk the olive oil, maple syrup and salt together in a small bowl. Add the cacoa powder whisking well until smooth.

Whilst the pears are still warm place 2 halves on each plate, pour sauce into the hollow of each pear.

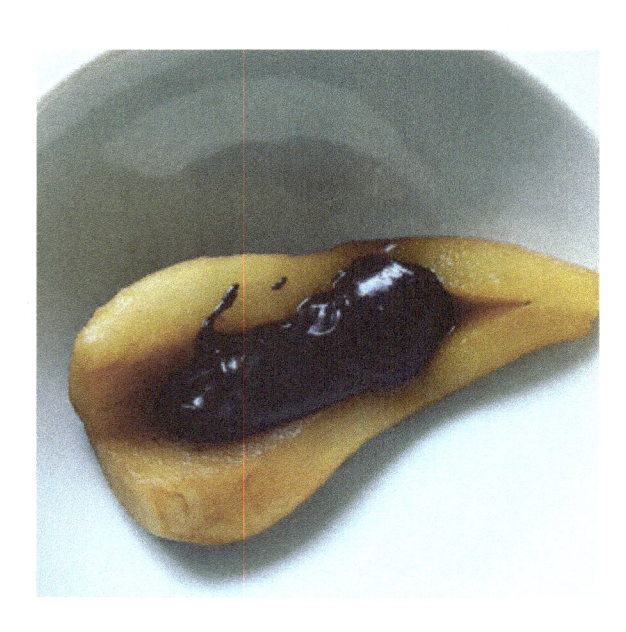

Index

Almond & coconut pancakes	23
Aubergine with miso dressing	40
Aubergine with tahini dressing	41
Avocado and tomato salad	58
Baked apples	106
Baked scallops	75
Beanotto with spinach	87
Berber eggs	5
Bircher muesli	14
Bissara broad bean soup	33
Bread maker gluten free bread	18
Buckwheat pancakes	22
Butternut miso soup with soba noodles	36
Cauliflower based pizza	93
Cauliflower rice	48
Cashew cheese	54
Chargrilled cauliflower salad	62
Chicken chimichurri	82
Chicken satay with vegetable noodles	76
Chickpea & feta salad	64
Chickpea & kale hotpot	90
Chia yoghurt pots	8
Chocolate avocado mousse	96
Chocolate red velvet cake	101
Coconut and chickpea curry	92
Coconut and lime salad	66
Courgetti with feta & herb pistachio pesto	63
Creamy berry porridge	15
Easy chicken stock	26
Energy balls	98
Fish and salsa parcels	71
Flapjack muffins	102
Flax seed crackers	19
Fresh spring rolls	53
Fresh tomato salsa	32
Gado gado	94
Ginger greens	50
Green smoothie bowl	10
Grilled figs	9
Grilled lamb with a herby salsa verde	81
Harissa whole roast chicken	85
Hazelnut and blueberry mini muffins	99
Home-made baked beans	24
Japanese salad	61
Kimchi pickles	44
Lemon berry muffins	103
Lentil, spinach and tomato soup	27
Light and easy Christmas pudding	100
Mangoes and pineapple in chilli syrup	107
Marinated turkey breast	79
Mexican black bean soup with fresh tomato salsa	31
Mexican spicy salmon	74
Mini ham and egg frittatas	4
Minestrone soup	37
Minute steak with chicory & rocket salad	83
Miso salmon with radish & courgette salad	70
Moroccan beetroot dip	39
Moroccan fish tagine	68
Muesli	13
Mum's chicken soup	26
My favourite chicken curry	80
Nigella's avocado and red onion salad	60
Nutty chocolate ice cream	97
Nutty granola	16
Nutty seed bread	17
Pear and fennel soup	30
Pink smoothie bowl	11
Poached nectarines with ginger cashew cream	105
Poached pears with raw chocolate sauce	108
Pomegranate, chickpea and mint salad	65
Prawn & tofu pad Thai	72
Quinoa burgers with tomato relish	88
Raspberry cashew cheese cake	104
Ratatouille	51
Roast chicken with butternut squash & sweet potato	84
Roasted butternut squash salad with Dukkah	57
Roasted butternut squash soup	28
Roasted red pepper soup	29
Roasted veggies	52
Salmon burgers with a fruity salsa	73
Sauerkraut	43
Scrambled eggs, smoked salmon & chives	2
Scrambled tofu	6
Smashed avocado with chilli & lime	20
Smoked fish paté	21
Spanish omelette	3
Spinach salad with sesame & tamari	59
Sprouted broccoli seeds	46
Sprouted seeds	46
Stewed apple	7
Sticky & spicy aubergine	42
Sweet potato wedges	52
Tarka dahl	47
Tempeh	45
Thai laksa with tofu & prawns	35
Tofu Pad Prik	86
Tom Yum soup with noodles	34
Turkey koftas with tahini dressing	78
Veggie bolognaise	91
Whole roasted cauliflower	49
Winter slaw	56
Yoghurt berry smoothie with walnuts & cinnamon	12

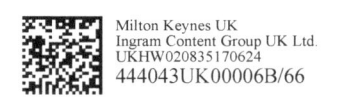